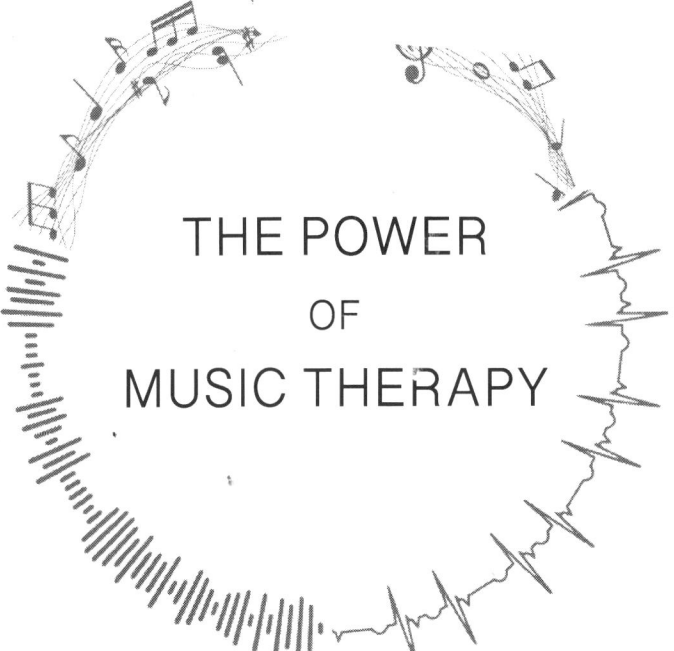

THE POWER
OF
MUSIC THERAPY

GILLIAN CUNNISON

The Power of Music Therapy
Copyright © 2023 Gillian Cunnison
All Rights Reserved
Paperback ISBN: 979-8-9895761-0-4 Ebook ISBN: 979-8-9895761-1-1

Cover design by the author

No part of this publication may be reproduced, distributed or transmitted in any form without the prior written permission of the author, except in the case of brief quotations.

The author made every effort to ensure the accuracy and completeness of the information contained in the book. These are her thoughts, ideas and memories from her objective and subjective perspectives and she has tried to represent events as faithfully as possible. The author makes no promise of results, expectations or experiences for the reader.

The titles of copyrighted songs are featured throughout this book.

Trademarked, copyrighted and registered terms mentioned throughout the book are listed below.

Boomwhackers®
Chord Buddy®
Chrome Music Lab & iGoogle Arts and Culture Lab from Google LLC™
Garageband™ from Apple Inc.™
Idiopan™
Incredibox®
InTandem™ (MR-001) by MedRhythms
LullaFeed™
Nordoff Robbins™
Pacifier Activated Lullaby System® by Powers Medical Inc. (acquired by NeoLight in 2022)
Relax Sounds from Matrix Software®
Rock Stix™
Soundtrap®

Neurologic Music Therapy Terms:
Melodic Intonation Therapy (MIT)®
Musical Speech Stimulation (MUSTIM)®
Musical Neglect Training (MNT)®
Neurologic Music Therapy (NMT)®
Oral Motor Respiratory Exercises (OMREX)®
Patterned Sensory Enhancement (PSE)®
Rhythmic Auditory Stimulation (RAS)®
Rhythmic Speech Cueing (RSC)®
The Academy of Neurologic Music Therapy®
Therapeutic Instrumental Musical Performance (TIMP)®
Transformational Design Model (TDM)®

To my Mum and Dad, for always encouraging
me to follow my dreams and for supporting
me wherever I am in the world

CONTENTS

Author's Note		6
Introduction		8
1.	I Am a Crocodile *Celebrating abilities with neurodivergent individuals*	19
2.	Ring of Fire *Initiating recovery after acquired brain injury and with veterans*	33
3.	I Believe *Developing coping skills in oncology*	46
4.	Sympathy For the Devil *Facilitating socialisation in group music therapy*	55
5.	Always a Star that Shines *Fostering self-worth in mental health*	65
6.	When the Saints Go Marching In *Increasing motor strength and endurance in physical rehabilitation*	74
7.	Stand Tall *Building resilience with children in adoption and foster care*	82
8.	Oh, What a Beautiful Mornin' *Reminiscing in dementia care*	90
9.	Pain Don't Hurt Me No More *Encouraging self-expression through songwriting*	101

10. No One Like You
Commemorating music for new beginnings and the end of life 112

11. Somewhere Over the (other side of the) Rainbow
Reflecting on some of the challenges of the profession 122

12. A Note to the Trainee Music Therapist
Giving some helpful tips and advice to trainee music therapists and anyone considering a career in music therapy 126

Concluding Thoughts 130

Resource List 134

Acknowledgements 141

References 145

About the Author 158

AUTHOR'S NOTE

This book is composed entirely of my own experiences which I hope will uplift and inspire others who read it. These personal accounts are purely from my own perception and the methods, interventions and techniques used are not necessarily the 'right' or only way to approach the situation. Furthermore, these are my experiences from training in the UK and working in the US. Music therapists from other countries may use different definitions, terms or ways of practicing.

The terms 'client' and 'patient' are used interchangeably throughout the book, depending on the setting. Confidentiality is of paramount importance in music therapy practice so names, and in some cases diagnoses, have been changed to preserve the anonymity and privacy of the individuals whose experiences or stories are included throughout. The only exception to this is for those who have kindly granted permission for their names to be shared in the book.

This book does not describe the intricacies of every step in the therapeutic journey for each story. Music therapists must complete an assessment session with every individual they work with and a treatment plan with goals and objectives is then written. Data is tracked and every session is documented in medical records or other relevant files. Adjustments are made within and between sessions and treatment plans and client goals are regularly updated. Often there is also a lot of preparation required before sessions such as finding resources or learning songs. When clients reach their goals or are discharged, a procedure for closure before termination is undertaken. Additionally, other daily and hourly tasks such as cleaning instruments after each session are carried out for the well-being of each client. While these steps are not detailed in the book, they constitute an integral part of the therapeutic process.[2]

Finally, given the significant number of people I had the privilege to work with over the years, it is neither possible nor practical to know the current circumstances of each one or where they are now. While some of the stories within this narrative do offer updates on the individuals featured, others do not. If, by chance, our paths have crossed and you happen to remember our time together, please don't hesitate to reach out—I would love to reconnect!

INTRODUCTION

Try to imagine a world without music. A party without music. Your favourite movie without its soundtrack or a workout at the gym without music. Significant moments in life without music—the first dance at a wedding in silence or a birthday celebration without singing "Happy Birthday".

Now think about how often you might have been surprised at yourself for singing along to lyrics you didn't think you knew at a concert or remembering a radio jingle or a theme song from a childhood TV show you hadn't heard for years.

This is the power of music.

Music is the only universal language that we can all communicate with, regardless of age, location or capability. It can activate almost all brain regions and networks (more than language) and can trigger the most specific of memories instantaneously. It connects us, inspires us and is always around us. For the past decade, I have been lucky enough to use the power of music to help countless individuals through my work as a music therapist. Every day I have been inspired by those I've worked with and their stories. I share some of these stories in this book and hope they inspire you too.

"Music is the great uniter. An incredible force. Something that people who differ on everything and anything else can have in common."[3]

- Novelist Sarah Dessen

What exactly is music therapy?

The first documentation of the healing capabilities of music dates back to as early as the times of philosophers Plato and Aristotle, around 380 BC.[4] There are also musical instruments that are said to be as old as human cave paintings.[5] However, it wasn't until the First and Second World Wars that musicians, teachers and bands began to play for wounded and traumatised soldiers with Post Traumatic Stress Disorder (PTSD) that the field of music therapy began to become more commonly known.[6] Today over 200 music therapy degree programs are offered worldwide and there are over 20,000 practicing music therapists globally who have undertaken an undergraduate or graduate degree in music therapy. This is then followed by an application to their country's regulatory body for music therapists and a requirement to maintain their certification through continuing education each year. Exact requirements vary by country.[*]

Music therapy is now defined by the American Music Therapy Association (AMTA) as

---

[*] Not all countries/areas worldwide have a regulatory body, certification requirements and/or continuing education requirements. You can refer to the World Federation of Music Therapy (WFMT) website (listed in the Resource List) for more information regarding specific countries. The number of music therapists is estimated using 2017 data from the WFMT.

> *"the clinical and evidence-based use of music interventions to accomplish individualized goals within a therapeutic relationship facilitated by a credentialed professional."*[7]

In short, music therapists use music, in all forms, to work on non-musical goals for each individual they work with, from birth to the end of life. The goals may be cognitive, emotional, physical, behavioural, communicative and/or psycho-social and can help to promote wellness, alleviate pain, manage stress, express feelings, enhance memory, improve communication and promote physical rehabilitation, to name a few. Following an assessment of each patient, often using assessment tools specific to the individual's diagnosis[†], a treatment plan is made and it is most commonly the case that multiple goals are worked on within each session for a specified amount of time. The ultimate aim in music therapy is to see these goals and skills transferred beyond the therapy setting. The evidence-based and goal-oriented nature of music therapy differs from other modalities such as sound healing, sound baths and sound wave therapy (which I also love to participate in!) as well as volunteer community music and listening to binaural beats.

In the following chapters (in no particular order), you will discover how music therapy manifests in reality and real individuals' lives. Each chapter includes information on a diagnosis leading into personal stories and music therapy journeys. The chapters are named after a memorable song in each respective journey.

[†] Examples of various music therapy assessment scales and tools are listed in the Resource List.

My story

Music has been a huge part of my life from a young age. I began learning the violin at the age of seven and piano at age ten, later followed by percussion in high school and guitar and ukulele in my twenties. I have vivid memories of discovering the brilliance and artistry of renowned classical music composers while learning the piano, often practising for hours on end. Chopin's "Nocturne Op. 9 No. 2" and Rachmaninov's "Piano Concerto No. 2" would give me goosebumps while I listened to them and even more so while learning and practising. I distinctly remember finding out about the complexity and intricacy of the works of Bach for the first time. Incredibly, his "Goldberg Variations" can be turned upside down and still yield a playable masterpiece[8]—a testament to the unparalleled genius of his penmanship.

During my childhood I also began to realise how important and iconic movie soundtracks are—themes from *Superman*, *Jaws, Jurassic Park, The Lion King, Titanic* and *The Piano* left a lasting impression on my musical journey. I also remember the exhilaration of hearing the band Aerosmith for the first time aged seven as "Walk This Way" blared through the speakers on the *Rock N' Roller Coaster* at Disney's Hollywood Studios in Orlando, Florida. Soon after this I began building an extensive CD collection and remember sitting for hours looking through every detail of their album covers. I had the privilege of attending concerts by some of my favourite bands for the first time, including Muse, the Foo Fighters and the Red Hot Chili Peppers. I stared in awe at my idols with the opening notes of my favourite songs sending shivers down my spine. It was during these moments I knew I was hooked on the power of music.

I spent my teenage years playing violin and percussion in school ensembles, orchestras and brass bands including the National Youth Brass Band of Scotland, Bon Accord Silver 'B' Band and Granite City Brass Band. The energy of almost thirty musicians playing together with gleaming brass instruments, resounding vibrations of the drum kit and timpani and the clashing of cymbals was second to none. I loved (and continue to love) the camaraderie of playing music with other musicians. As musicians know, making music with others is truly special and unique and the deepest bonds are often made. Even for those who don't make the music, people will always bond over shared music interests, music festivals and concerts until the end of time.

I have also always been passionate about the medical field and caring for others, so in my final years of secondary school in Scotland I began the long and arduous process of applying to medical schools and was proud to secure a place at the University of Aberdeen. In the summer between high school and university, aged seventeen, I travelled to India to complete a two-month volunteer project in an orphanage and hospital in the southernmost state, Tamil Nadu, to gain more experience in the caring and medical fields. During this time, however, I became very sick with an unidentified stomach virus and upon returning to Scotland to begin medical school, the virus returned multiple times during my first semester. Faced with a heart-wrenching decision, I reluctantly chose to withdraw from the program and take the remainder of the year out, despite the extensive effort it had taken to secure admission. I now know that the universe works in mysterious ways, however, as it was during this time that I found out about the field of music therapy. What had initially been a period of great disappointment transformed into excitement when I realised I could combine my two passions—music and medicine—with a career in music therapy.

I earned an undergraduate degree in music in 2009 including an exchange year in Sydney, Australia and a master's degree in music therapy in 2013. I then moved to the US, completing additional fieldwork and an exam to become a board-certified music therapist (MT-BC). Since music therapy is a relatively small field, a lot of dedication, patience and many hours of applications were required to secure work. My first contract was only four hours a week at an acute rehabilitation hospital, setting up a new music therapy program to treat brain injuries, spinal cord injuries and strokes. I was fortunate that the hours gradually built up as word spread about how beneficial music therapy was for their patients. In the meantime, I gained other invaluable experience in many different settings through additional contracts including private practice, in schools, memory care and with adults with developmental disabilities.

I have encountered many setbacks and difficulties throughout my career. Financially it has always been a struggle since most music therapy jobs are reliant on funding grants and underpaid for the level of education required. Still, I am incredibly grateful and feel fortunate to have had the opportunity to use the power of music therapy to help individuals through my work for the past ten years.

Catching the travel bug

It wasn't just a stomach bug I'd caught during that first trip to India. I was also bitten by the travel bug and I haven't stopped since! I am incredibly fortunate to have now travelled to 54 countries, gaining many unique experiences along the way while travelling on a shoestring budget. I have realised more and more over the years that the majority of people I meet around the world have never even heard about the field of music therapy or their understanding is limited to thinking that it is listening to music through headphones or learning an instrument. I have lost count of the times I've heard the response to asking about what I do for work—"That's cool. What is it? I've never heard of it!"

In light of this, three years ago I decided to set out and write about a few memorable experiences out of hundreds over the years that I thought others would enjoy reading about and perhaps be inspired by, while learning a little bit about the benefits of music therapy. Fast forward to now and I realise parts of this book have been written in California, Florida, New York, North Carolina, Ecuador, Mexico, Nicaragua and Scotland. I have thought of sections to add while on planes, trains, ferries, in cars, on bikes, on walks, in the gym, at the beach and even while surfing. Something I quickly learned while writing this book is that you never know where or when writing inspiration is going to strike!

In the following pages, I share the stories of some incredible souls who have made and continue to make a significant impact on my life, both professionally and personally. I am proud to share them and I am forever grateful for their permission to do so.

Music therapy in action

For music therapy patients, live music-making creates amazing and unique opportunities. I had the honour of seeing a patient being motivated to move his arm for the first time to shake a maraca after sustaining major debilitating injuries in a car accident. I saw a cystic fibrosis patient's face light up as bright as a pair of Rockstix (motion-activated LED light-up drumsticks). I witnessed a veteran with PTSD increase his self-esteem after creating a new rhythm on a djembe drum. I watched a whole family bond and laugh while playing colourful Boomwhackers together after their loved one's major surgery, which required an extended length of stay in the hospital. I was lost for words when a patient with aphasia after an acquired brain injury, unable to say her name, sang lyrics from The Beatles' song "Hello, Goodbye" clear as a bell. A teenager with cerebral palsy smiled for the first time in days after hearing the soothing ring of a tone chime and the quiet composure of a burn patient as she was comforted by the music during the procedural support for her dressing change all remain poignant memories for me.

Every day I am inspired by those I work with and can see first-hand how music and sound uplift and rehabilitate those who need it most. A few years ago, I used an Idiopan (sometimes called a 'tongue drum' or 'happy drum') to provide vibrotactile feedback for a toddler with a hypoxic brain injury. The instrument's vibrations and tuning to a C major pentatonic scale eliminating dissonance ('clashing' sounds) are especially calming for patients. I have also used the same instrument during procedural support for a teenager with complex medical needs while EEG monitoring leads were placed on him in the epilepsy monitoring unit. For this patient, the sound and vibrations were mesmerising. It completely distracted him from the pressure of the leads being glued to his skull and the chemical smells of the glue itself, which can be an overstimulating procedure. I have calmed an infant by laying her on top of a huge gathering drum and letting her gently feel the steady rhythm throughout her body. This rhythm is soothing for infants since it is reminiscent of the mother's heartbeat in the womb.

Songwriting and recreative music also play a significant role in music therapy. Through song, feelings are often expressed more easily, particularly to those who struggle with self-expression. I have seen a patient with global developmental delay freestyle rap for almost ten minutes straight and witnessed a little girl sing using the most meaningful metaphors despite refusing to talk at home. Songs can increase self-esteem, communication, confidence and self-expression after setbacks and help build resilience. They can also tell stories of pain, hopefulness, the future, relationships and heartbreak—the list goes on.

Thank you for reading!

I hope this book will be a small snapshot into the world of music therapy and that the stories resonate with you. This book is for anyone who enjoys music, is interested in discovering more about music therapy and how it can benefit others, is interested in exploring music therapy for themselves or their loved one(s), or who may just enjoy reading an inspirational story. For the training music therapist, I hope this helps to see what 'a day in the life' might be like for you! In addition, although anonymous, some individuals referred to in these chapters would not have the chance or the ability to share their own stories. I wanted to write this book to share the stories and words of those who don't have a platform for their voice.

Thank you for reading this book and taking the time to learn about these wonderful people to gain a small glimpse into the world of music therapy. If you liked reading it, please share! I would love to play a small part in helping to spread the word about what music therapy can do. If you would like to know more or if you know someone who you think might benefit from music therapy, please get in touch!

Find me on social media: @gillian_cunnison

Or through my website: www.telemedmusic.com

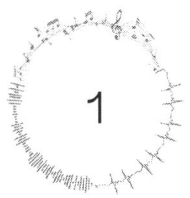

I AM A CROCODILE

Celebrating abilities with neurodivergent individuals

"Where words fail, music speaks."[9]
                         - Author Hans Christian Andersen

The term 'neurodivergent' describes people whose brain variances influence their cognitive processes, resulting in distinct strengths and challenges that diverge from those without such variations. This term encompasses a range of conditions including medical disorders and learning disabilities. Among these are autism spectrum disorder (ASD)[‡], attention-deficit/hyperactivity disorder (ADHD), Down syndrome and epilepsy, as well as chronic mental health illnesses such as obsessive-compulsive disorder (OCD), bipolar disorder and borderline personality disorder. The significance of neurodivergence lies in rec-

---

[‡] Autism spectrum disorder is the official medical definition of autism, but many autistic people and families feel that the term 'disorder' is too negative for everyday discussions and that autism is a difference rather than a disorder. The words autism and autism spectrum are also widely accepted by autistic people. I use the preferred terminology for each individual I work with, however I use the official medical definition ASD throughout this book.

ognizing and honouring the unique ways in which neurodiverse individuals perceive and interact with the world, fostering a more inclusive and accepting society.

Disabilities and exceptional abilities

So often, I have seen first-hand that with disabilities come exceptional abilities. I've lost count of the number of times I have been left speechless by individuals I have worked with who have been labelled in society as being neurodiverse yet with naturally impressive skills and, more often than not, they are entirely unaware of how impressive they are! Molly, a talented drum student of mine and now also a friend who is diagnosed with Down syndrome, never fails to recite any musical theatre or Disney song lyric word for word during our sessions. Danny, diagnosed with ASD, knew the entire Beatles anthology by heart by the age of eight when I worked with him and is now an outstanding steel drummer with the ability to play a blues scale at record speed.[10] Talents often stretch far beyond the realm of music, too. Daniel, also diagnosed with ASD, excels as an exceptional skier and has a unique gift for remembering dates. He can tell you what day of the week any date—past or future—falls on and the year any Disney movie was released. The story of British artist Stephen Wiltshire serves as another striking example. His ability to create a nineteen-foot drawing of New York City's sprawling skyline in photographic detail from memory after only a short helicopter ride over the city[11] is also a testament to the astonishing potential within neurodiverse individuals.

Neurodiverse individuals often get overlooked or underestimated when it comes to their talents. However, neurodiversity often gives individuals a unique lens through which they view the world and helps them create in ways that might outshine others. The way music seems to 'unlock' hidden strengths or abilities buried deep within souls can appear magical. For scientists, the mystique of music's power continues to captivate and there is much more to be discovered about precisely what makes our brains so susceptible in response to its allure.

In the context of autism, the daily marvels witnessed by music therapists resonate with research on what is known as mirror neurons—specialised components of the brain that spark to life when we observe another person execute an action.[12] Imagine watching a friend pick up a pencil and begin writing; the mirror neurons in our brain have the same response they would exhibit if we were holding the pencil in our own hand. The theory is that these mirror neurons function differently in people with autism; thus, they imitate from their own point of view.[13] This difference potentially contributes to their struggles in empathetically connecting with others' emotions, interpreting and decoding social cues and easing into the back-and-forth rhythms of verbal conversation. These very skills are the ones that music therapy nurtures. This nurturing is grounded in the elemental facets of music-making—imitation, repetition, pattern recognition and non-verbal communication—all of which have a transformative impact on the brain regions that diverge in structure for people with autism. These insights illuminate the synchrony between music therapy's interventions and the areas in

The music child

The term 'the music child',[14] coined by Paul Nordoff and Clive Robbins in 1977, refers to the belief that even amid the challenges of disability and trauma, an innate facet of well-being resides within the individual that can be awakened and engaged with music. I saw this philosophy in action when volunteering at the Nordoff-Robbins Center for Music Therapy in Manhattan, New York, for the summer of 2010. Within the sessions led by music therapists Alan Turry, Michele Schnur Ritholz and Jaqueline Birnbaum, the profound connection between the therapists and their clients during their sessions bore witness to this principle—truly tapping into and connecting with each client's inner being, fostering a remarkable bond and transcending the barriers of disability and trauma.

My time in New York inspired me to delve further into the Nordoff-Robbins approach and enrol in a master's degree at Queen Margaret University in Edinburgh. Central to the Nordoff-Robbins training program lies improvisation, harnessing the harmony, melody and rhythm elements of music to "cultivate self-awareness, discipline, self-expression and concentration within each individual".[15] This music-centred approach[16] is firmly grounded in championing abilities over disabilities, celebrating the unique potential residing within each person and combining the concept of 'musicing'. Musicing is the act of "listening with reverent attention".[17] For example, if a child is shrieking, that could form the start of a melody. If a child is rocking back and forth, that is a steady beat that can be used in the music. As a result, individuals who might seem uncommunicative can actually express themselves in their own unique way through the music. With music-centred improvisation, therapists can also use the music accompaniment to 'unstick' clients who are stuck in a rigid way of playing, first by meeting the client where they are at in the moment with the music (what is known as the iso-principle) and helping them to transition to something different.

Singing before speaking

"Music may be the activity that prepared our pre-human ancestors for speech communications and for the very cognitive, representational flexibility necessary to become humans."[18]

- Daniel J. Levitin in This is Your Brain on Music: The Science of a Human Obsession

At times, especially for children, singing comes more naturally than talking. Some children I have worked with sing constantly, rarely using their speaking voice at all. From a very young age, music mnemonics (using rhythmic-melodic templates for rehearsing verbal information) are used to facilitate the recall of verbal information. Cast your mind back to the familiar melody of the "ABCs" or the playful repetition of "Head, Shoulders, Knees and Toes" you learned as a child. These early musical encounters exemplify the memory-enhancing capacity of music. Music is structured, repetitive and predictable, particularly in children's songs, naturally facilitating word retention, which is helpful for those grappling with cognitive challenges. Repetition is vital for development and memory, significantly contributing to the enduring popularity of songs. This sometimes makes for a little extra patience, however—perhaps when the umpteenth rendition of "Baby Shark" plays on the TV!

An intriguing fact also emerges when exploring the interesting phenomenon of singing and speech. Numerous speech impediments, including stutters, vocal tics and even Tourette Syndrome, often disappear while singing. Researchers at The University of Iowa delved into this realm and found that as music activates the right hemisphere, distinct from the left hemisphere responsible for language processing, singing essentially shifts the cognitive process.[19] Consequently, the left brain's tendency to trigger stutters and impediments is bypassed during musical expression. This intricate interplay between music and language offers a window into the human brain's complexity, highlighting music's potential to foster remarkable transformations.

Structured vs. unstructured experiences

As previously mentioned, music is effective in children with neurodiversity because it is structured and predictable. Often, sessions have the same format, starting and ending with a hello and goodbye song to frame the session—providing familiarity and comfort. However, for some individuals with neurodiversity, it is more beneficial to have much less structure. So often, other aspects of life (including school with rules and routines) are structured;

therefore, being in a room and having a connection with someone rather than being told what to do, without barriers, where they can completely be themselves and have their own voice through the instrumentation, is more effective. In this case, the music therapist would often follow the client's lead (known as a 'client-led' approach), perhaps starting with musically reflecting the client's responses to their environment. After this assessment, various instruments and interventions can be introduced to see what motivates or excites the client (or equally what does not interest them) and the session continues from there.

Our senses and how they play a role

Did you know that we have seven senses? While hearing (auditory), sight (vision), smell (olfactory), taste (gustatory) and touch (tactile) are widely recognized, two additional senses are essential components of our perceptual experience: vestibular and proprioception. The vestibular sense governs our perception of movement and motion, facilitating our ability to navigate smoothly, while proprioception pertains to our body awareness and understanding of our physical position in space. Some of these senses can be overloaded or underloaded for children with neuro diversities, leading to sensory sensitivities. Here, music therapy interventions emerge as an impactful avenue, helping to regulate sensory experiences and provide opportunities for sensory integration in an organic way through an accessible and engaging medium.

Playing a single song with an instrument will activate multiple senses. For example, the song itself will provide auditory input. Adding a cabasa—a small hand-held percussion instrument constructed with loops of steel ball chain wrapped around a cylinder with a plastic handle—rolled on arms and legs will add visual, tactile and proprioceptive inputs. If the child is on a scooter board while doing this, we also target vestibular input. But the sensory journey doesn't end there. Other non-musical items can also benefit—scarves sway, body socks cocoon, weighted blankets soothe, stretchy bands engage, wobble boards challenge and bean bags provide comforting weight. These items are especially beneficial for children who require extra input to feel their bodies, which is common in individuals with ASD. When paired with music, these items become instruments of sensory exploration, enhancing the therapeutic journey with textures, weights and movements that target proprioceptive and vestibular needs. In short, all of these layers combine to transform this single song into a whole sensory experience.

Additional items can also be included in interventions for additional input if appropriate including puppets, letter boards, pinwheels, toy animals, music-related board games and bubbles. There really is no limit to a music therapist's bag of tricks! It also doesn't have to be complex—even clapping hands to a rhythmic stimulation is an example of sensorimotor integration and dancing to music without looking at our bodies demonstrates kinaesthetic perception.[20]

Music can be used to calm the body if it is dysregulated. Breathing exercises or songs with a slow tempo and gentle cadence can serve as effective tools to help regulate and manage the nervous system, guiding the body back to a state of equilibrium. This is particularly helpful for diagnoses such as dysautonomia, an umbrella term used to describe different medical conditions that cause a malfunction of the autonomic nervous system. Music and the nervous system are linked to the sensory system, also explaining the phenomenon of frisson—music giving us goosebumps.[21] Frisson happens when a sound wave hits the cranial nerve, signals then fire, and the thalamus is lit up.

Songs and songwriting can help children understand and express what their body needs at that moment—or maybe even just that they need a break. As music therapists, we also adjust our musical output in the moment according to the sensory system and how our clients are feeling, attuned to the sensory landscape of our clients. We might compose a song in the moment, perhaps transition to delicate fingerpicking on guitar (making a much softer and gentler sound than strumming), or even re-tune the guitar to open-D (DADGAD) tuning, creating an airy and familiar sound.

In essence, music becomes a mirror for many neurodivergent children, a medium through which they explore their identities and roles within the world. It provides a space for self-discovery, expression and understanding, nurturing the profound journey of self-awareness and connection for each unique individual.

Training the brain

Music doesn't only stimulate our senses; it is almost like a brain workout. While listening to music, our brains simultaneously process hearing, melody, timbre, pitch, emotion, volume, movement, beat perception, relative pitch, harmony and sequencing.[22] For a simple task of playing an instrument within music therapy, a child could also be working on:

- Joint attention and increased attention to a task
- Note/colour/letter identification
- Improved cognitive functioning
- Decision-making and executive functioning skills
- Sequencing
- Cause and effect relationships
- Improved behaviour
- Decreased agitation
- Increased socialisation
- Decreased self-stimulation
- Improved receptive/expressive language
- Successful and safe self-expression
- Improved self-confidence, self-esteem and/or self-worth
- Improved gross motor, fine motor and/or sensorimotor skills
- Enhanced auditory processing

A recent study at the University of Bath also showed that playing the piano boosts brain processing power and helps lift the blues.[23] Another study at the University of Chichester found that 90 minutes of drumming per week helped adolescents with ASD overcome hyperactivity and attention deficits.[24] Learning drumming patterns also tunes brain connectivity in areas associated with inhibitory control and self-regulation.[25] I am continually thankful to researchers for scientifically proving what I see on a daily basis, as music therapy is often considered an additional or non-essential treatment and not given the same funding or insurance coverage as other therapies. My hope is that this will change in the future with further evidence-based research.

Liam and the crocodile

I met Liam while working at a small school for neurodiverse children. He was five years old and diagnosed with ASD, OCD and selective mutism, an anxiety disorder characterised by a person's inability to speak in certain situations or social settings. In Liam's case, this manifested within the school environment, leading to his lack of response to teachers and peers. He was also very particular with food at school and home, as is often the case with children diagnosed with ASD, OCD and/or ADHD.

Our sessions began with instrument exploration, developing the therapeutic relationship by building rapport and ensuring Liam felt comfortable. He would follow directions well, seamlessly navigating colour-coded notation on the keyboard and even following song actions with precision. However, there was never any speaking or singing. I felt helpless—all I wanted to do was help him find his voice.

During one session I introduced a children's song "I am a Crocodile" to him and he enjoyed crafting little castanet crocodile instruments to play along with the music. The first verse unfolded:

> *I am a crocodile, long and strong*
> *And some little monkeys won't leave me alone*
> *They've gotta be careful; they've gotta be kind*
> *Otherwise I will...bite!*
>
> Copyright Ahjay Stelino

Liam's enthusiasm for the climactic 'bite' ending was evident. Laughter, delighted squeals and the snap of his castanet crocodile converged, exemplifying his joy. Then it happened. During one rendition of the song, he said "bite!" A single syllable that carried so much meaning and defied all expectations. The feeling I had was indescribable; I couldn't believe he had filled in the word so clearly and on cue. I was so proud. With each subsequent session we worked more on the song and, slowly but surely, he filled in more words I had left a pause in my guitar accompaniment for. Finally, he was singing the whole song!

Soon, the end-of-term showcase came along. The showcase was an event for all students to perform to parents and caregivers something they had been working on throughout the year, taking centre stage to present the fruits of their year-long endeavours. By this point, I had prepared Liam for his moment over several weeks and his unwavering participation throughout our sessions was an assuring testament to his readiness. However, the dynamics shifted significantly as he now faced an audience brimming with anticipation and expectation—a whole different ball game.

I shouldn't have worried. Liam recited the whole "I am a Crocodile" song word for word, with the correct cues, in the right moments, and with extra expression and enthusiasm at the end! I truly couldn't believe not only his participation but his newfound confidence. Music had become his safe space and, despite his world being so overwhelming, he could finally share this space with others.

The audience was also impressed. After the showcase, one teacher at the school wrote:

> *"I'm speechless!! Liam shined so brilliantly. In turn, you provided his family with such a gift—a type of gift they do not often get—to revel in the wonder, talent, and sheer joy of their child. In this moment, they could put aside worry, frustration, and perhaps guilt and just be proud parents."*

Support in the outside world

The neurodivergent individuals I have worked with hold a special place in my heart. Fortunately, this feeling is shared across the globe, generating a lot of support in so many ways with a multitude of supportive initiatives. Advocates for neurodiversity have diligently championed the cause, spotlighting the benefits of inclusive theatre groups, workplaces and arts groups to name a few. Sensory-friendly concerts and events extend a welcoming hand to neurodiverse individuals, offering solace through noise-dampening headphones or allowing occasional respites in dedicated break rooms when suffering from sensory overload.

On a personal note, the privilege of working with neurodiverse individuals has been enriching and humbling and has taught me so many invaluable insights. They illuminate the beauty of the present moment, navigating life's challenges with an unwavering positivity that serves as a beacon of inspiration. Through them, we can see life's true treasures, transcending the monetary and materialistic pursuits that often preoccupy us. The essence lies in the radiance of shared joy and finding a lesson given by those who greet each moment with an authenticity that resonates deeply within us all.

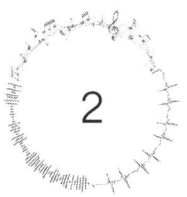

RING OF FIRE

Initiating recovery after acquired brain injury and with veterans

"I regard music therapy as a tool of great power... because of its unique capacity to organize or reorganize cerebral function when it has been damaged."[26]
— Neurologist and author Oliver Sacks

In 2011, US Representative Gabby Giffords was targeted during a violent shooting spree at a public constituent meeting event in Tucson, Arizona. The attack resulted in the loss of six lives and injured twelve others. Gabby was shot through the head, sustaining a traumatic brain injury that necessitated years of dedicated rehabilitation. She attributes a substantial portion of her recovery to the music therapy she received at Houston's TIRR Memorial Hospital, having to relearn to speak after the gunshot tore through the left side of her brain.[27] While the traditional pathways for speech were compromised, Gabby's journey highlights the impressive adaptability of the brain. Areas critical to speech are situated in the left side of the brain but, even if they are damaged, it is possible to 'retrain' the other side of the brain (where more musical processing happens) to take over. Neurologic Music Therapy (NMT) serves as a vital tool for this, offering a range of effective techniques, including:

- Melodic Intonation Therapy (MIT): sung or chanted melodies resembling natural speech intonation are combined with tapping to improve speech independence and fluency

- Rhythmic Speech Cueing (RSC): a rate-control technique using auditory rhythm either in metronome form or within music to cue speech

- Musical Speech Stimulation (MSS): the last word of the phrase of a well-known song is eliminated to stimulate non-propositional speech, literally 'pulling out' the words

Studies have shown that participants show notable improvement in language functions even after one session of Melodic Intonation Therapy[28] and that the percentage of intelligible speech increased from 65% to 89% through Rhythmic Speech Cueing in patients with severe speech deficiencies.[29]

Neurologic Music Therapy was developed by music therapists Michael and Corene Thaut, founders of the Academy of Neurologic Music Therapy. The foundation of NMT is based on the Transformational Design Model (TDM)[30], which is used for designing clinical protocols. There are six steps to TDM:

1. Assessment of the client's strengths and needs using an initial assessment and pre/post test
2. Develop goals and objectives
3. Design non-musical interventions for goals
4. Make the non-musical interventions musical
5. Reassessment
6. Transfer the client's progress to functional life skills

Essentially, the premise of NMT is using music as a tool with the end goal of increasing a required skill.

Promoting functional language

Song lyrics are valuable tools used by music therapists for many reasons you will see throughout this book. During sessions with brain-injured patients, they are used in Musical Speech Stimulation to promote functional language—the language we need to communicate in different day-to-day situations. After complete language loss from a brain injury, the focus narrows on cultivating the vocabulary essential for heartfelt connections with loved ones. This aims to restore the vital bridge of communication that sustains human relationships, signifying the core of music therapy work.

Some of the most well-known songs that have been enjoyed for decades are surprisingly the most powerful. As I continued building my ever-growing music therapy 'toolbox' by learning more and more songs tailored for specific situations and patients, I realised how interwoven the lyrical narratives of many songs are with our everyday encounters, circumstances and experiences.

For example, The Beatles' song "Hello Goodbye", as mentioned in the Introduction, incorporates the words *hello, goodbye, yes, no, stop, go, why, oh no, I don't know, high and low*. Eleven of the most important functional words and phrases are conveniently placed within a few song lyrics, complete with prompt words for the therapist—"You say …" and "I say …" Thank you, John, Paul, George and Ringo!

The Jackson 5 song "ABC" incorporates letters (A, B and C), numbers (1, 2 and 3) and three solfège syllables (Do, Re and Mi). The full solfège scale—Do Re Mi Fa So La Ti Do—comprises seven of the most popular syllables used in English-speaking countries.

"Rock Around the Clock", made famous by Bill Haley & His Comets, also incorporates numbers in sequence from one to twelve, with number repetitions in each verse.

Depending on the severity and nature of the injury, we may even start with something as simple as forming vowel vocalisations, such as the opening 'ahh's' in ABBA's "Dancing Queen", then eventually work up to words and phrase formations.

The list of useful phrases, words and letter formations, including different categories, is endless. A few examples are shown in the following table. One thing is for sure—I never thought of music and lyrics in the same way after my music therapy training!

Days of the Week	Numbers
Happy Days - TV Show Theme Song	9 to 5 - Dolly Parton
	7 Years - Lukas Graham
Feelings	**Phrases**
I Got You (I Feel Good) - James Brown	I Just Called to Say I Love You - Stevie Wonder
Happy - Pharrell Williams	Survivor - Destiny's Child
Letter formation -B	**Letter formation - D**
Barbara Ann - The Beach Boys	Banana Boat (Day-Oh) - Harry Belafonte
Build Me Up Buttercup - The Foundations	Zip-a-Dee-Doo-Dah - from Disney's Song of the South, performed by James Baskett
Letter formation - E	**Letter formation - L**
Take it Easy - The Eagles	Brown Eyed Girl (Chorus) - Van Morrison
Easy on Me - Adele	Piano Man (Bridge) - Billy Joel
Letter formation -M	**Letter formation - N**
Stand by Me - Ben E. King	Hey Jude (End Section) - The Beatles
Lean on Me - Bill Withers	Na Na Hey Hey Kiss Him Goodbye - Steam
Letter formation - P	**Multiple letters spelling**
Poker Face - Lady Gaga	L-O-V-E - Nat King Cole
Paradise City - Guns N' Roses	Respect - Aretha Franklin

Work in rehabilitation has brought some of my favourite and most memorable moments over the years. Among these—seeing a loved one's face light up as they hear a 'hello' greeting from the hospital bed for the first time, especially in the wake of a transformative life event, is profoundly unique and priceless—highlighting where the intangible magic of music transcends words and imparts an invaluable connection.

Edwin's journey

Edwin spent his whole adult life in the army from age eighteen. He had been deployed all around the world, including Germany, Haiti and Iraq. Thirty-one years of dedicated service culminated in 2013 and he was ready to enjoy his retirement.

Fate chose a different course, however. During his final deployment as a sergeant in Afghanistan, aged forty-nine, Edwin's path was irrevocably altered after he sustained a devastating traumatic brain injury from detonating an Improvised Explosive Device (IED) on a minefield. He was transported back to the US to start full-time rehabilitation. The abrupt transition from the disciplined routine of military life to the confines of a medical facility immediately posed an immense emotional and psychological hurdle for Edwin. Then, another cruel blow. Shortly after starting his rehabilitation journey, he suffered a stroke[§] as a result of the initial brain injury.

I began working with Edwin in 2016. At this time, he had trouble walking and needed to use a cane and a notable slur characterised his speech. He wore sunglasses due to his eye being cut by shrapnel. His whole left side was weak. He had difficulty remembering and forming words combined with blurry vision and his sustained concentra-

---

[§] Also referred to as a cerebrovascular accident (CVA)

tion was limited to only five minutes before he succumbed to a splitting headache. Despite these hurdles, struggles and adversities, Edwin always entered the sessions with an infectious smile and was ready to work! In his tall and robust frame resided a calming, gentle soul, embodying kindness and patience—a true definition of a 'gentle giant'. His presence was a bright light and he was a true joy to be around.

Around the same time our sessions started, a significant addition to Edwin's life unfolded. A service dog, Liberty, was organised to be gifted to him as a surprise from his wife through the Patriot Military Family Foundation. Liberty quickly became a loyal companion and sidekick who accompanied him each week.

Rocking out

Edwin loved all music, especially classic rock, and was interested in learning the guitar. I decided we would begin with the ukulele, a more accessible instrument for learning, thus an effective bridge to learn the guitar. I sourced an adaptive guitar pick with an extra rubber loop that wraps around the thumb to help with grasp so it didn't fall while we worked on strumming. We also started working on his gross motor arm strength and coordination through djembe drumming, alternating the right hand and left hand. We would play slow at first then slowly increase the tempo. We addressed Edwin's fine motor strength using the lap harp—a small trapezoidal-shaped harp with simple notation sheets slipped under the strings, making it easy to follow.

The weeks went by. We played other calming percussion instruments while singing, such as the rainstick. I implemented the NMT speech rehabilitation techniques of Melodic Intonation Therapy and Rhythmic Speech Cueing to pace and slow down each word to increase clarity. I introduced visual and reading goals for Edwin, visually tracking modified chord charts and lyrics to songs on the keyboard. For cognition, I used a sequence of different rhythms on different instruments, each with its own rhythm to remember. We practised singing and playing at the same time—a challenge in itself for anyone. We also talked about Edwin's memories of songs that he listened to while on deployment such as Johnny Nash's "I Can See Clearly Now" and the Tracy Chapman classic "Give Me One Reason". The lyrics are poignant in these two songs with themes of hope, courage, overcoming adversity, resilience, reasoning and heartbreak.

The months then went by and after working together for a year, Edwin's progression was evident. From his initial struggle with maintaining focus for just five minutes before needing a break, his concentration increased to a full hour without headaches. He reported that he could move his fingers more easily and quickly and his left arm also required less effort to move.

In addition to all the cognitive and physical goals that Edwin benefitted from in music therapy, he also appreciated the structure in his day, mirroring the regimented routine he had long been accustomed to during his time in the army. It was also a positive appointment among the continuing medical appointments at the VA hospital and the support and camaraderie developed in our client-therapist relationship were equally beneficial for him. The sessions significantly enhanced his mood and he would look forward to coming each week. As did I! He was the longest and most consistent patient I had worked with and we developed a close bond. I won't forget the profound connection that unfolded as Edwin's journey evolved and flourished.

In 2019, thanks to the efforts of his dedicated care worker, Sheri, Edwin was gifted a brand-new acoustic guitar through a grant from the American Patriot Music Project—a non-profit charity based in California supporting veterans through music. Edwin loved his new shiny blue guitar and was so proud of it. He was also able to attend 'Warrior Weekends' through the Wounded Warrior Project. Warrior Weekends provide a weekend of rest, relaxation and fun for heroes who have injuries sustained while serving on military duty with their spouses and families, at no cost to the participants. After the Warrior Weekends, I could feel a wonderful sense of renewed energy and pride in Edwin.

We began working on the same adaptive chord charts as I introduced guitar chords, first using a Chord Buddy—a revolutionary device that affixes to the neck of the guitar with each button creating a different chord structure. With time and practice, his progress reached a significant milestone, graduating to form the chord shapes independently, unassisted by external devices.

The first song we played together with Edwin playing independently on the guitar was Johnny Cash's "Ring of

Fire", using the chords we had learned first—G, D and C. The guitar is a difficult instrument to pick up for anyone, never mind someone with so many hurdles to cross. What a testament to Edwin's strength, determination and dedication! This moment will always remain in my memory.

Edwin's own testimonial about his sessions is stated below.

> *"I feel good when I come here. My brain is learning something new. To me, music is very soothing. It relaxes my brain and I don't think about anything else. It has helped my confidence and my concentration has increased. I have the ability to learn how to do different things with the guitar and ukulele that I didn't know how to play before."*

I had the honour of working with Edwin for four years. COVID-19 restrictions sadly ended our sessions together, but I am also happy to note that Edwin is still receiving music therapy services in the community through Piedmont Music Therapy based in Charlotte, North Carolina.

Continuing work with veterans

My work with veterans continued and guided me towards working on additional goals besides neurologic recovery, encompassing mental health and addressing post-traumatic stress disorder (PTSD) through lyric analysis and songwriting. Interestingly, for the veterans I worked with, the genre they connected to the most was country music. While this preference posed a unique challenge for my own personal growth as I was not the biggest fan of country, I quickly recognized that the transformative nature of the stories of many country songs is highly beneficial for veterans, allowing them to connect on a deeper level. Often in life, if someone hears of a story of hardships similar to theirs and the storyteller manages to get through that struggle, it is easier for the recipient of the storytelling to relate, perhaps use that story to work through their own journey, find solace within shared experiences or even just to know they are not alone in the struggle.

The process of overcoming challenges, as depicted in these songs, often translated into a relatable source of inspiration. Together we looked at themes such as anger and its effect on relationships in Tyler Childers' "Shake the Frost", loneliness and journeys in Jason Isbell's "Traveling Alone", resilience and starting new chapters in Chris Stapleton's "Starting Over", and developing a supportive network in "Better Together" by Luke Combs. With these themes and stories and through exploration, each veteran was also inspired to craft and share their own versions, transforming their personal stories into melodies of empowerment.

This genre challenged me, but hand in hand with challenge comes opportunity. I had the chance to empathise with hardships that diverged starkly from my own reality—which I will hopefully never face in my own life—through the eyes of others. Through the narratives woven by these artists, I witnessed their profound impact on the lives of individuals with whom I had the privilege of working. It was truly a transformative and humbling experience and in turn I also developed a newfound appreciation for country music. In hindsight, this challenge was a gateway to many invaluable insights and for that, I will remain forever thankful.

In their own words

It has always meant so much to me when hearing from patients I have worked with, in their own words, how music therapy and our time together have benefitted them. These testimonials authentically unveil the impact of music therapy—one can never know the true impact until it is heard from the patients themselves first-hand.

Allow me to share two examples of individuals with acquired brain injuries who exemplify the spirit of hope, perseverance, courage and the ability to transcend adversity. These narratives encapsulate the essence of this chapter as it draws to a close.

> *"I learned so much from you and I believe my speech improved. I gained the confidence to speak again and my hands are more flexible. I just realized no one hangs up on me anymore and when I call friends and family, we have conversations and I think they understand most of what I say by what they reply. You are so talented, so caring, and you went way beyond anything I have experienced before. Thank you."*

> *"It gave me confidence that I can speak again in front of strangers which I had lost. I never dreamed I would sing again in front of anyone. I now realize I can be accepted as me. I did not believe that. I thought I would never be accepted unless I was as I was before, which you and I both*

know will never happen. I didn't really believe that I could be whole again (the new me). I wanted to believe it, but I was not there yet. I will work harder than ever, but now it gives me a real reason to do it. I can begin to heal and accept myself."

3

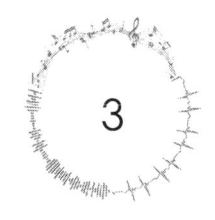

I BELIEVE

Developing coping skills in oncology

"Music was my coping mechanism. I could place myself out of my body. It humbles you."[31]
- Musician Kelly Price

For oncology patients, music can be an outlet for expression and hope. It can be a safe place for patients to explore fear, anxiety and anger—the range of emotional responses to living with and battling cancer. It can help by offering a distraction from medical procedures while alleviating pain and reducing anxiety.[32] Simultaneously, it can bestow invaluable coping mechanisms, nurturing and building skills requisite to cope with a patient's new diagnosis, their new reality and environment.[33] Through developing these skills, patients can take control of their hope within the throes of the most critical health circumstances. Moreover, the physiological impact has been shown in the form of the boost of protein levels that combat microbial infection[34], lowered levels of the stress hormone cortisol and improved quality of life overall.[35] Singing also releases dopamine, the 'feel good' hormone.

Music therapy is powerful and effective despite being non-pharmacological (not using medications or other chemical interventions). That being said, the importance of a trained music therapist is paramount since profound emotions very often rise to the surface. In these instances, the music therapist's training and experience guide them on how to effectively navigate these emotions in the moment and process them with the patient while ensuring the patient feels safe and supported.

Remembering the caregiver

The caregiver is sometimes forgotten about or overshadowed in oncology, particularly in the modern medical landscape. However, supporting the caregiver is very important, for they often bear the brunt of the long and difficult experience. Music therapy can not only assist in navigating challenging emotions but can also benefit the caregiver by helping them process difficult emotions and relieve the stress that accompanies burnout. In certain instances and, when deemed appropriate, music therapy sessions together with the patient and caregiver can also help foster connection and communication.

The work of Dean Quick, a dedicated music therapist at Levine Cancer Institute in Charlotte, North Carolina, is a testament to this. He has worked with cancer patients and their caregivers for many years, facilitating collaborative songwriting and recording ventures. I remember one particular serendipitous encounter—meeting Ginny, the wife of one of Dean's former patients, who was coincidentally a neighbour of a friend of mine. Upon finding out I was a music therapist, she immediately burst into a heartfelt tale, reminiscing about how much it meant to her to be able to listen to the recordings she and her late husband Val had made together before he passed.

Charlene's journey

I knew that Charlene was special from the moment we met. She was beautiful yet modest. She was engaging with piercing, intense eyes yet had a calming aura. She was also very sociable, always chatting with anyone who passed by her room.

Charlene had been diagnosed with leukaemia seven months before we met and had just completed another round of chemotherapy when we first started sessions. While collaborating with her care team, it was decided that increasing her coping skills was a priority. In our first session, she reminisced about playing the piano throughout her childhood—an ideal entry point for our musical journey. Choosing something a patient is familiar with is often an effective way to start sessions, as it makes the patient feel comfortable and more in control.

We began improvising on the black key pentatonic scale, using only the black keys of the piano. As mentioned in the Introduction, this scale eliminates any dissonance or 'clashing' notes, thus creating a very peaceful and relaxing sound. This is also a very accessible and easy way to introduce or reintroduce the keyboard, as there are no 'wrong' notes to play. We would also use the Dorian mode, characterised by its blend of the natural minor scale with a major fifth, evoking a simultaneous moody yet uplifting sound. When paired with a repeated low 'D' drone note, this mode gives the music a grounded and safe feel.

These improvisations often went on for a long time. Afterward, Charlene would express that it felt like an escape for her to get lost in another world without anxiety, stress or her diagnosis, leaving her liberated within an alternate reality of harmonies and melodies.

She also loved to sing, particularly empowering songs by female artists. Among her favourites was "Brave" by Sara Bareilles, where she would take great pleasure in belting out the uplifting chorus. Another was the energising "Rise Up" by Andra Day about perseverance, courage and confidence, and Rachel Platten's "Fight Song" with its rallying lyric phrases. As I accompanied her on piano, guitar or ukulele, our collaboration forged a space where her voice could soar. With these two songs, Charlene could show the world she was brave, courageous and a fighter.

Her absolute number one and most beloved artist was Alicia Keys—with whom she shared an uncanny physical resemblance—especially the song "Girl on Fire". She would say that she could feel the music running through her veins whenever she was singing it and it made her feel alive, like her soul really was on fire. It was heart-warming to see her lost in the music, singing at the top of her lungs with her eyes closed. These visceral experiences transformed her, breathing life into her spirit and igniting her existence with vibrancy. I remember at the time finding myself wishing that all these artists knew the positive impact their songs had on Charlene, infusing her days with renewed zeal and elevating her quality of life.

Sometimes, we would also practise experiential music together with improvised lyrics following each other's lead, which often resulted in fits of laughter. As they say, and I believe it to be true, laughter is the best medicine! At times when she had more energy and wanted to move more, we would also drum together using small African djembes. She often said the lively rhythms would "wake her up and feel alive". Her sessions often followed the iso-principle, a concept previously mentioned in Chapter 1. The iso-principle is the process of the therapist matching a patient in their current mood state with the music, then gradually changing the music to help the patient shift to a different mood. The iso-principle can also be used to affect physiological responses such as heart rate and blood pressure.[36]

In moments when the weight of reality would become overwhelming for Charlene, I would use guided imagery scripts along with improvisations to create an immersive experience, helping her retreat into the 'other worlds' she enjoyed visiting in her mind. Guided imagery—using a script of words combined with music, which complements and enhances the writing—emerged as a powerful and beneficial tool, especially to regulate overwhelming emotions. One such example she particularly enjoyed was a script tailored around the theme of letting go, imagining emotions taking form as drifting clouds, slowly dissipating into the expanse of the sky. The musical accompaniment I provided, ranging from arpeggiated music on the keyboard to the ethereal resonance of percussion instruments like wind chimes and a glockenspiel, worked well to assist with these images.

There were also sessions where Charlene would succumb to a lot of physical pain. In such instances, I would facilitate a technique known as Progressive Muscle Relaxation, a sequential exercise involving the deliberate tension and subsequent relaxation of each muscle group in the body, usually from the head to the toes or vice-versa. This practice carries the capacity to alleviate muscle tension and, in turn, can be successful in distracting the patient from pain. Charlene would complete a numerical rating pain scale (1-10) before the exercises and the number she gave afterward would always be lower, sometimes only by one, sometimes by a bigger margin. Once we had completed this cycle of muscle relaxation we could then progress to gentle stretches and movements to the music, helping to ease her body from the tension of lying in the same position for prolonged periods of time.

As the weeks passed and her pain became more frequent, Charlene also found breathing increasingly difficult. This was due to a combination of anxiety and physical damage to her lungs from her medication and surgeries—the previous year she also had to have a tracheostomy tube placed in her throat. In response, our therapeutic trajectory shifted, channelling its focus toward breath support. The structure of music lends itself seamlessly to this, as breath support exercises can be used easily with the music supporting the tempo. One such technique, commonly known as square breathing, exemplifies this, involving inhaling and exhaling for equal durations, most commonly spanning four counts. This parallels the structural underpinnings of music, where sequences also often revolve around the four-count framework.

At Charlene's request, we increased her sessions to three times a week. Typically in our sessions, Charlene was creative and bubbly, often offering a lively exchange of anecdotes about her favourite things including art, music and Olive, her cherished tabby cat companion. Yet, there came a series of sessions where I sensed a shift in Charlene's spirits and she seemed more reserved and introspective. I asked her if she had been doing anything different in recent days, which might account for this change in mood. She disclosed that she had been channelling her thoughts into writing poetry and had also started journaling. She reached over to her bedside cabinet and retrieved a small leather-bound book from the drawer. Charlene was very open and enthusiastic about sharing these words with me without any prompting or requests, flipping through the pages and reading some of her writings out loud. The raw eloquence of her prose, including phrases like *I believe in the girl in the mirror, I'm taking control* and *I can still be myself,* painted a portrait of her resilience and determination. It was so inspiring to hear these uplifting words and phrases from someone going through so much.

I suggested we write a song together using her words, offering to set them to music. She eagerly agreed. I rearranged the poem and set it to a melody. Her poetry evolved from ink on paper into an emotional and powerful ballad. Below are the lyrics of the finished song, "I Believe":

I believe in the girl in the mirror
I believe in me, you and I
I believe in myself
You can't take it away

Chorus
I believe, I believe, I believe
It's not my time to go, I'm alive
I believe, I believe, I believe
Anything can happen
I'm taking control

No matter what happens
I can still be myself
It's the truth
You can't take it away from me

It's okay what you're feeling
You're not the only one
You find confidence in yourself
I have the courage and the strength

The resonance of Charlene's message, characterised by its unadorned simplicity and profound authenticity, has stayed with me throughout the years. This positive mindset got her through the most arduous and challenging times. Throughout our sessions, I witnessed the ebb and flow of her emotions, most often culminating in a brighter, elevated mood as our time together drew to a close each session. Charlene's journey resonates with me still, a journey that has shaped not only my practice but also my approach to guiding others. Even if they have never ventured into this realm, encouraging patients to journal their thoughts has become a cornerstone of my therapeutic philosophy—a tribute to the transformative power of words and the depths they can unearth. Try it yourself. You never know what might come from it and how it might impact you!

Charlene and I had developed a close bond during the time we spent together. As I reflect on her treatment program, I am reminded of just how much we accomplished in sessions and how each of the interventions helped her cope in that particular moment. Each intervention, carefully tailored to the unique cadence of her emotions and experiences, was a vital coping mechanism guiding her through her health journey. The end of our time together led to creating a tangible memento—a recording of "I Believe". She loved the recording and listened to it daily.

A few weeks later, Charlene was discharged from inpatient to outpatient oncology services. Shortly after this, I moved to a new state. I was happy to hear after I moved that Charlene had achieved complete remission. Tragically, however, her leukaemia returned and she passed away a year later.

Charlene's legacy resounds and I often think back to her strength. As I recall her journey, I am reminded of her courage and how hard she fought. She was a true inspiration and motivated me to volunteer the following two summers at Camp Happy Days, an incredible organisation providing free week-long residential summer camps for children with cancer and their siblings in South Carolina.

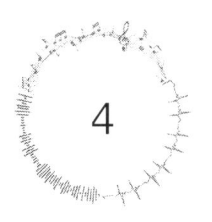

SYMPATHY FOR THE DEVIL

Facilitating socialisation in group music therapy

"Bringing people together is what music has always done best."[37]

- Journalist and writer Rob Sheffield

It is a well-known fact that music brings people together. We hear it at every party, gathering and events of every size and scale. Its absence would make the world a very quiet and lonely place. In addition, hospitals and other medical institutions can be incredibly isolated environments and making music can be highly beneficial to combat loneliness. Multiple studies have shown that loneliness and lack of social contact with others can diminish healing, increase stress and anxiety and negatively affect the way the immune system functions.[38] In 1955, when he was thirteen years old, George Harrison from The Beatles decided he wanted a guitar of his own while hospitalised at Alder Hey Hospital in Liverpool for inflamed kidneys.[39]

One can't help but wonder how different the music world may have been had this experience not kickstarted his musicianship!

The live music effect

Musical vibrations, though intangible to the tactile senses, possess an incredible ability to traverse the entirety of the human body. Suppose you are in a concert hall or a stadium—here you will feel the vibrations differently and more intensely than when listening to music through headphones. In such immersive environments, the sensations are heightened compared to the cocoon of headphones. The Scottish virtuoso percussionist Evelyn Glennie, who has been profoundly deaf since the age of twelve, feels the vibrations of music through her bare feet while performing on stage. She is an incredible performer and was my original inspiration to pursue learning percussion after participating in one of her workshops in the North East of Scotland aged fourteen.

English broadcaster and author Fearne Cotton eloquently describes a particularly memorable moment while seeing iconic British rock band Queen perform live in her book *Bigger Than Us:*[40]

> *"Bohemian Rhapsody clung to my ears and made my heart race and my feet prance."*

Think back to the exhilaration you felt seeing your favourite artist in concert or the emotions and pride rushing through you at your child's first school recital. Think of the high-spirited sounds of gospel singers, church choirs or live bands connecting with the souls of religious congregations. There is a scientific reason for this. When we hear a song we like, it activates a dopamine release in our brain as the sound wave lights up different receptors.[41] Additionally, in 2016, a study conducted by researchers at Imperial College in London proved that multiple sets of concertgoers experienced decreases in cortisol (the body's primary stress hormone) and other stress hormones.[42] They did so at a greater intensity than previously studied subjects who listened to non-live music. What I thought was particularly interesting was that the age and sex of the participants, their musical ability, nor their familiarity with the music being performed didn't seem to matter.[43] The power of music travels unanimously across every board. Using psychometric and heart-rate tests, a study of live music concert-goers also found that a participant's well-being increased by 21% after just 20 minutes of concert attendance, compared to a 10% increase after participating in yoga and 7% after dog walking.[44]

Thankfully for all of us there is no shortage of live music across the globe and now that pandemic times are behind us, it's back and here to stay. Likewise, countless organisations and groups worldwide provide opportunities to embrace and lift up communities through the arts (although, unfortunately, most are underfunded). I certainly know that I wouldn't be the music therapist I am today without all of the school orchestras, musical theatre productions, bands, community music events and other arts organisations I have been a part of throughout my life. Music (and the arts in general) challenges us and opens our minds. As musician Pete Townshend from the English rock band

The Who once said, "the day you open your mind to music, you're halfway to opening your mind to life."[45]

I also love to hear the inspiring stories and watch performances shared online of community groups and organisations providing solidarity at times of hardship, including grief choirs, fundraising drum circles and orchestras for children in the poorest areas of the world, to name a few. These organisations are the true definition of sharing experiences and building community to lift each other up in times of need.

Tapping in

In music therapy, the job of the music therapist is to 'tap into' each individual's abilities, to write non-musical goals for each patient and to challenge the patient; however, it is imperative to tread cautiously, steering clear of excessive demands that can lead to decreased motivation—the opposite desired effect. Another common role of a music therapist, particularly in group settings, is to support what is already there in the music and add in what is missing to shape it. This might mean providing a supportive beat, a bass line, a harmony or maybe something more percussive. Equal inclusion for each client in group music therapy is hugely important, as well as structuring the task for the level (cognitive, emotional and physical) of each group member—all while making sure all of the exercises are welcoming.

Music therapy sessions are often one-on-one due to the nature of each patient's individualised goals but there are many times when group music therapy is even more beneficial for the patient, especially when considering the invaluable social dimension it introduces. If you are lucky as a music therapist, you might also have the opportunity to co-treat (also known as 'joint working' in the UK) with other therapists. Interdisciplinary collaboration is most helpful and music therapists benefit from the expertise of each respective field (including art therapy, child life, chaplaincy, counselling, dance movement therapy, healing touch, occupational therapy, physical therapy, recreation therapy and speech-language pathology) for collaboration on assessment, advice on a clients' symptoms, treatment plan ideas and co-treats.

Assembling the band

One particular group music therapy session, my very first as a board-certified music therapist, will always stay with me. For this session, I was the lucky one to have the opportunity to co-treat with Christina, the manager of inpatient speech pathology therapy and original creator of the music therapy program at Kessler Institute for Rehabilitation. Let me set the scene.

Three patients who were all in the hospital for very different reasons were selected for the group after we had worked with each patient individually first. Two were musicians and one had not touched a musical instrument since childhood. However, a common thread uniting them was their love of music, a passion that ignited their motivation and enthusiasm to join the group. There were many roadblocks and hurdles to overcome to get the group together when faced with ever-changing medical schedules and the patients themselves often not feeling good or not having enough energy for the group. With time and a lot of coordination, we finally had everyone together and we were ready to make music!

On the left, a 17-year-old boy, Jason, had accidentally fallen off a cliff while riding his bicycle and was undergoing rehabilitation for paraplegia from the waist down. He had been learning the drums before his accident. Jason loved playing them and talking about his favourite songs to play along to. In the therapy room, he was setting up an adaptive drum kit we had created for him in his previous individual music therapy session. This kit required only upper-body movement and included congas, cymbal, cowbell, tambourine and an adapted bass drum he could play with his hands. Jason had been working hard with the kit in his sessions to strengthen his core and arms and in his previous session he had been able to push himself in his wheelchair for the first time since his accident.

In the middle was Harry, a 47-year-old professional jazz saxophonist. Harry had been recording tracks in a music studio in Manhattan when he suffered a stroke, now presenting with total weakness on his left side. We began working on regaining the strength in his left arm and hand by playing the metallophone (an instrument similar to a glockenspiel but with a deeper, softer sound). At first, Harry expressed uncertainty and doubt about his ability because he was unable to successfully grasp the mallet to play the instrument. A quick collaboration with his occupational therapist resulting in some medical tape strapped around the mallet and his hand easily solved the problem, however!

On the right, Michael, a 55-year-old patient diagnosed with locked-in syndrome—a devastating rare disorder of the nervous system that completely paralyses the whole body with the exception of the muscles controlling eye movement. The 2007 biographical drama *The Diving Bell and the Butterfly* beautifully represented this diagnosis. Essentially, the patient is locked inside their own body and the long-term prognosis unfortunately doesn't usually see a lot of change. However, on rare occasions, some movement is regained and Michael was fortunately one of these exceptions. Through rigorous therapy, he had managed to successfully 'unlock' some independent arm movement and was now able to play the keyboard with his forefinger. Michael was a huge fan of music—particularly the Beastie Boys and other 80's punk—the true British definition of a 'muso.'

We decided to start with a song everyone was familiar with, which included a driving rhythm for the percussionists. The chosen debut song was the Rolling Stones' "Sympathy for the Devil". In my opinion, this is a true masterpiece of a song and a great start for the group because of the repetitive nature of the backing instrumentation. Everyone knew their part from the previous individual therapy sessions we had facilitated and all of the group members were excited for it to come together.

Cue Jason's congas intro and we were off! (If you haven't heard this song before, listen to it now, you won't regret it!) One by one, Christina and I went round to each group member to assist in adding their part to the layers of sound before adding our own instruments—guitar and flute, as well as the iconic "woo woo" backing vocals. Everyone became completely immersed in the rhythm and the music. The atmosphere in the room was so electric it gave me goosebumps. Against all odds this group was jamming, and jamming hard! I will never forget the glances shared between the group members—all complete strangers thirty minutes prior—who were bonding and connecting through the music. We kept this jam going for quite a while, at times improvising over the top of the rhythm. It was apparent we were causing quite the scene because, by the end of the song, we had a whole audience watching at the door!

About a week later, we received this message from one of the hospital's executive team members, who had been following Michael's progress.

"Seeing Michael sing and play today brought tears to my eyes. I want to thank Christina and Gillian for all the amazing work and dedication in progressing him with his rehab goals and reconnecting him through the power of music. I was so proud to see this program truly come to life and through the context of such a complex patient."

We were thankful for this acknowledgement and we were proud of ourselves, too. This was the first time we had created a group of this nature after an intensive three months dedicated to building a brand-new innovative music therapy program at the hospital. We had achieved a milestone. This time was also poignant for me on a personal level, as this was precisely what I had worked hard for during my master's degree training. Finally, being able to create these opportunities for others in need was becoming a reality. We had many more memorable jams in the following weeks until the patients were discharged from inpatient rehabilitation a few weeks later.

Continuing the momentum

We continued facilitating groups whenever possible and when we had the means and resources. The intricate nature of many patients' needs often necessitated hand-over-hand assistance, so we were sometimes limited by the number of therapists available. We also ran groups specifically targeting speech rehabilitation goals multiple times a week.

We soon realised that no hurdle was too big for us to overcome regarding a patient's physical limitations. The premise of the Neurologic Music Therapy technique TIMP (Therapeutic Instrumental Musical Performance) means that almost any instrument can be adapted for a patient, regardless of the complexity of their injuries or diagnoses. We enjoyed thinking out of the box about how to adapt the instruments in our growing collection. We had tambourines strapped to patients' feet, paddle drums flying high and low to encourage stretching and movement and kazoos, harmonicas and recorders to encourage breath support and control (often ending in infectious laughter!).

I have been fortunate that my journey has led me to facilitate many other groups throughout my career, including a detox unit for substance abuse, a rehab unit in a children's hospital, skilled nursing and memory care facilities, a teen behavioural health unit, an arts centre for adults with developmental disabilities, groups for toddlers and teens with Down syndrome and whole class sessions in schools. Although the patients and environments have differed vastly, the theme has always remained the same for these individuals—a resounding commonality across all the experiences is that music can connect and support people in a way no other medium can.

5

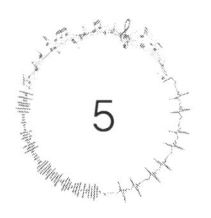

ALWAYS A STAR THAT SHINES

Fostering self-worth in mental health

"Mental health is a lot like the ocean. It swells and subsides. It comes and goes. It rises and falls. And everyone's rhythm seems to be different."[46]

— Writer, coach, podcaster and former pastor Steve Austin

We are now, unfortunately, living in a global mental health crisis. The United Nations has predicted that the COVID-19 pandemic has caused a 25 to 27 percent increase in the prevalence of depression and anxiety around the world.[47] In adolescents, recent statistics from the US Centers for Disease Control and Prevention (CDC) are even more shocking—a team of researchers found an increase of 73% in suicidal attempts by poisoning in children aged ten to twelve in 2021 compared to 2019[48] and a study in 2023 showed that an alarming one-third of teenage girls in the United States have seriously considered attempting suicide.[49]

In the current age of social media, which has brought immense social pressure including comparing ourselves to others, it is too easy to slip into a constant state of self-loathing. Music can help us to look inward and encourage self-esteem. It can lift us up when we are down and comfort us when we are having difficulties. As mentioned in Chapter 3, music therapy can holistically provide all of this without chemical intervention. By no means am I diminishing the importance of modern Western medicine, but this is significant in the current medical world where potent medication drugs are readily available and often over-prescribed—especially in the United States.[50]

Identity and sense of self

> *"In the social jungle of human existence, there is no feeling of being alive without a sense of identity."*[51]
> - Psychoanalyst Erik H. Erickson

The specific role of music therapy for adolescents with mental health difficulties is commonly considered with particular emphasis on identity and the self.[52] Dealing with the emotional rollercoaster of adolescence is a complex process and some teenagers may struggle to emerge from these years with a coherent sense of who they are. In this sense, identity refers to a person defined by their circumstances, family, peers, experiences and emotional state. A crisis of identity is an integral part of adolescence, without which the sense of self (how you perceive yourself as a whole) may not be as firmly established. However, often identity crises take the form of anxiety which manifests as having difficulty in consolidating a sense of self, often leading to withdrawal from school and social and family contact and eventually requiring professional help.[53] For people whose sense of self is fragile, where meaning is lost or not easily found, music has unique and extraordinary properties that music therapists can use to support integrative processes of becoming or finding connections or meanings in order to thrive with self-confidence and self-assertion.[54]

Developing a strong identity and sense of self can also lead to positive self-assurance around others. The Outburst Project is a music therapy program for LGBTQIA+ individuals in Nottingham, England.[55] One participant in the project had experienced bullying at school, depression and social anxiety, which stopped him from wanting to sing. Outburst helped him to express his personality, make new friends and consider a career in music. He stated the following while reflecting on the program.

"I'm more sociable, outgoing and self-confident now. If I hadn't gone to Outburst, I would probably still be wallowing in self-pity and feeling like I don't have any friends. Singing helps me tell people about the challenges I face."[56]

Trauma and music therapy

Researcher and professor Hanoch Yerushalmi at the University of Haifa in Israel asserts that an individual's ability to adapt their coping skills to a traumatic situation can determine either an outcome of growth or of stagnation.[57] Many individuals with differences experience trauma, not as we know it, but in their own ways because they are not understood. In another case study, music therapy helped a patient "appreciate his unique qualities" and deal with "feelings of being an outsider in the harsh social environment of middle and high school".[58] No matter what stage of life or troubles, we want to give a space to express, reflect and enable young people to forge a path to self-acceptance.

Ashleigh's journey

I began working with Ashleigh in a behavioural health unit to which she had been involuntarily admitted after a suicide attempt. She was fourteen years old at the time and had been previously diagnosed with an eating disorder at the age of twelve.

Initially, she was one of the most testing patients I had worked with as she was very resistant. She was not trusting of others and I didn't blame her—from reading her medical history, she had been exposed to abusive relationships throughout her entire childhood. In a world where she had been let down time and time again, it was only natural that her guard was firmly in place—a barrier to protect herself from further harm. Collaboration with the behavioural health care team enabled me to primarily develop goals to decrease her anxiety and increase her self-worth, commonly addressed with mental health and eating disorder diagnoses.[59]

Introducing music therapy can cause uneasiness or apprehension for individuals like Ashleigh and there is a good reason for this. Researchers found that musical or athletic performances and speaking to adults were two of the most anxiety-inducing situations for adolescents.[60] I know first-hand what this is like after suffering from crippling stage fright for many years despite learning and performing music from the age of seven. It would be so severe that all I would be able to see during a performance was blurry and jumbled music notes on the page. Stepping into the spotlight, through music or any other avenue, can open up strong emotions and involuntary reactions.

It is also essential to use instrumentation appropriate for the client's age from the first introduction of services. Young children usually engage well with small, colourful, shiny instruments, but it is best practice to use full-sized instruments with teens and adults so that the person doesn't feel inferior or think that the therapy is childish. Of course, we are lucky to now also have technology at our fingertips.

Like most teenagers in her generation, Ashleigh loved technology. I therefore had an easy and inviting way to introduce her to music and begin to develop trust which is of utmost importance in the therapeutic relationship. We began with the GarageBand app, Launchpad app and the website Soundtrap—all excellent and effective apps for creating and expression. Thankfully, they are all very user-friendly, using pre-composed loops, sounds and digital instruments. I would guide her through as she engaged in fitting together each track, creating new and unique compositions.

Other apps and websites we used are listed with their descriptions below.

Chrome Music Lab	A website that makes music more accessible through fun, hands-on music and sound experiments.
iGoogle Arts & Culture Lab	A website database offering easy and fun ways to get creative with sound through various arts projects from all over the world.
Incredibox	An app that lets you create your own music with the help of a "merry crew of beatboxers". It is almost like a video game, where you can drag and drop sound icons on different characters to make music. The player can find combos to unlock animated bonuses and record mixes to integrate a ranking.
Relax Sounds	An app where you can design and mix ambient sounds and music to create your own relaxation tracks.

After trying these out and exploring all they had to offer, Ashleigh developed a newfound openness and was more accepting of new ideas in the session. She said she felt ready to try some live instrumental playing. I introduced the Idiopan first, mentioned previously in the Introduction. Sometimes called a 'tongue drum' or 'happy drum', the Idiopan is a metal circular drum tuned to the C major pentatonic scale, eliminating 'dissonance' (clashing notes), thus creating an extra calming effect when played to help decrease anxiety. We spent a lot of time improvising and exploring the soundscapes with the Idiopan. I then introduced the Q Chord, an instrument incorporating technology from a basic keyboard and electric guitar, combining both in a portable casing with a strum plate, a rhythm section and a chord button section. She loved exploring the different sounds, chords and accompaniments and singing along with the backing beats. We also worked on the ukulele donated by the Ukulele Kids Club, an organisation that provides free ukuleles to children in hospitals.

By this point, I was happy that Ashleigh and I had developed a healthy therapeutic relationship and felt ready to challenge her further with her growth. We moved on to a lyric analysis intervention, first talking about the song "Feeling Good Like I Should" by Sunday Best. One line of lyrics alludes to everyone having tough times but trusting that everything will work out; another addresses feeling overwhelmed and encourages personal grounding. This song offered the opportunity to discuss self-worth, resilience and strength and provided her with the structure and opportunity to process her own thoughts in an engaging way. By evaluating her own responses, Ashleigh was also able to increase her self-awareness.

After analysing other artists' lyrics, Ashleigh expressed a desire to narrate her own story. This also helped facilitate a sense of control which would help her cope with feelings and other situations. Feeling out of control is common in eating disorder and other mental health diagnoses, resulting in the patient using other behaviours to negate this.

The songwriting began. Her first song, "Always a Star That Shines", was exceptional and memorable. I was impressed by the skilful way she shared all her vulnerabilities, struggles and difficulties while leaving room for hope and positivity to shine through—all in one song.

Verse 1:
She was just a little girl
Living in her fantasy world
Trying to do what is right
Make the best of life
She turned away from all her dreams
When she hit 13
She felt like she couldn't do anything right

Chorus:
But there's a time when we all find
There's always a star that shines brighter than the other
One that can see the world but in color
Forever and ever
Would be tougher than the other
But the future is bright for one
A beautiful star that shines
Oh a star that shines beautifully tonight

Verse 2:
She's looking back
At all of her dreams
Trying to find the meaning
Why did all her dreams just stop
Making her keep wondering
She felt as if she was all alone
But then her perfect song came on
And she sang

We collaborated on recording the song and Ashleigh shared the recording with a few people around her in the unit. Sharing the recording proved instrumental in allowing them to understand her feelings and ultimately made her feel less isolated. Her care worker and nursing staff also reported marked improvements in her ability to manage her emotions and engage in social interactions.

Through technology exploration, instrumental improvisation and songwriting, music therapy provided opportunities for Ashleigh to not only express herself but also increase her self-worth and build healthy relationships. I hope that it continues to do so for millions more people in need. Ashleigh was discharged from the unit a few weeks later to an outpatient facility and it is my hope that she made use of these newly developed skills as she navigated through the last of her teenage years.

6

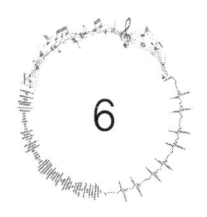

WHEN THE SAINTS GO MARCHING IN

Increasing motor strength and endurance in physical rehabilitation

"I wanted to prove the sustaining power of music."[61]
- Musician David Bowie

In 2010, a sports psychology study revealed that listening to motivating music enhances physical performance during exercise and delays fatigue.[62] Other studies have shown that songs with higher beats per minute (BPM) can also make us move faster and raise our heart rate.[63][64] For centuries, people have been motivated to work by music—songs and chants have historically propelled laborious tasks through generations. It makes sense as our bodies are naturally rhythmic and intrinsically motivated by rhythm; our hearts have a rhythmic beat and we walk to an internal rhythm. From toe-tapping to head-bopping, rhythm is an intrinsic part of our existence.

Music and physical rehabilitation

These facts also explain why the benefits of music therapy are not limited to the cognitive. As highlighted in previous chapters they can also be physical, using this natural internal musicality to facilitate movement while motivating clients to cope with treatment and the healing process. An otherwise monotonous exercise repeated every day (slow and steady repetition is key in rehabilitation) can be more fun and diversified with the addition of music. Moreover, when someone is in need of physical rehabilitation, it likely means they have been through some form of trauma. Music can help patients feel more relaxed and comfortable with their therapist, especially when combined with the reassuring familiarity of music they already know.

In music therapy sessions with physical goals, music can be specifically targeted to rehabilitate patients with many diagnoses including Parkinson's disease, dementia, stroke, cardiac and pulmonary patients, spinal cord injuries and visual deficits, including spatial neglect. Neurologic Music Therapy techniques used for this include:

- Patterned Sensory Enhancement (PSE) which elicits movement with musical cues through elements of music, including tempo, rhythm and dynamics. One example is a 'sit-to-stand' movement, which can be created by using an ascending broken piano chord cue since the action we are trying to facilitate is standing up.

- Therapeutic Instrumental Musical Performance (TIMP) is playing instruments, not necessarily in the conventional way, which exercises and stimulates functional movement patterns. For example, paddle drums can be placed at either side of the patient to cue stretching movements (and core strength) from side to side.

- Musical Neglect Training (MNT). Patients with a brain injury can also experience a deficit in awareness, as if the space opposite to their lesion in the brain does not exist anymore, known as 'neglect'. It is most common to have neglect on the left side following an injury to the brain's right side. One example of this is using desk bells arranged in a musical scale. While playing the scale of C (C-D-E-F-G-A-B-C), the brain 'predicts' the end of the scale located in the neglected zone. Another example is placing an instrument in the hand of the neglected side and a mallet in the hand of the healthy side (requiring the patient to cross the midline over to the neglected side), thus retraining the brain to recognise this side.

- Rhythmic Auditory Stimulation (RAS) is based on rhythmic and repetitive auditory stimuli. It uses external rhythm in the form of a metronome or recreative music to facilitate internally generated rhythmic movements such as walking. A Cochrane review of seven studies showed RAS can improve gait-related issues such as stride length, gait velocity, cadence and symmetry.[65] Extensive data significantly suggests that music therapy has positive impacts on walking patterns in patients with Parkinson's disease.[66]

- Oral Motor Respiratory Exercises (OMREX) are facilitated to improve articulatory and respiratory control using small wind instruments such as kazoos, harmonicas and recorders, as mentioned in Chapter 4. Patients with COPD (Chronic Obstructive Pulmonary Disease), asthma and other respiratory disorders can also benefit tremendously from music therapy to increase breath support and stamina. Simply increasing the length of musical phrases can help to increase lung capacity, resulting in increased breath support.

When clinicians and researchers used music therapy in stroke and gait disorders, they also discovered that music elicited movement.[67] They noted reduced impairments in the patients' limb movements and improved sensory impairments. Overall, an improvement in health was observed in the stroke patients group compared to the control group who didn't receive music therapy.

Further benefits in the physical rehabilitation world

Additionally, on June 30th, 2023, MedRhythms reached a significant milestone with the listing of InTandem (MR-001) with the U.S. Food and Drug Administration—a first for a technology leveraging principles of the neurologic music therapy intervention, Rhythmic Auditory Stimulation.[68] The Class II, prescription-only medical device is designed to be used by patients at home and is indicated to improve walking and ambulation for people with chronic stroke. MedRhythms, a company based in Maine is led by Co-Founder and CEO Brian Harris, a board-certified music therapist and neurologic music therapist fellow.

Time after time, session after session, I have seen patients make incredible progress with the addition of music. It is nothing short of awe-inspiring to witness. What's more, patients often have so much fun playing with the instruments that they sometimes forget they are even in therapy!

As the world-renowned neurologist and author Oliver Sacks stated in his book *Musicophilia: Tales of Music and the Brain,*

> *"Music can lift us out of depression or move us to tears - it is a remedy, a tonic, orange juice for the ear. But for many of my neurological patients, music is even more - it can provide access, even when no medication can, to movement, to speech, to life. For them, music is not a luxury, but a necessity."*[69]

I truly believe in this quote and have been lucky to see its truth before my eyes, one example being Libby.

Libby's road to recovery

I met Libby while working in an acute physical rehabilitation hospital in 2015. It was January and the rehabilitation team had learned that her family home had burned down during the night after a faulty Christmas tree light sparked and set their Christmas tree on fire. Libby and her two brothers were forced to jump from their second-floor bedroom windows to escape the blaze that quickly spread throughout the house. Instantly, their lives changed from thriving high schoolers—playing sports and being active members of their school's marching band—to sustaining spinal cord injuries and severe burns. Their long road to recovery began.

At only seventeen years old, Libby was a testament to intellect, radiance and quick wit. Conversations with her revealed a love for learning and dreams of attending university and travelling the world. Despite the devastating and traumatic upheaval that had completely changed her life's trajectory, Libby's positivity and determination remained steadfast.

One of Libby's primary rehabilitation goals was to increase her standing endurance. Her spinal cord injury had reduced her ability to stand independently for more than two minutes in her physical therapy session without rest, even with back support from her physical therapist. Her therapy sessions were both frustrating and exhausting for her.

Since Libby was a trombone player, a co-treat was arranged with her physical therapist to use her instrument as a motivating force. I collated some of her favourite songs that she had played with her school marching band and arranged them for trombone and piano. We began to play and again we soon witnessed the magic of music. Libby was so focused on playing that she would forget that she was standing! All of a sudden, more than six minutes had passed without any back support at all.

Libby enjoyed her music therapy sessions so much that we doubled the frequency of sessions, recognizing their transformational impact. I arranged more of her favourite band songs for myself on piano and Libby on trombone while adding two more musicians—the manager of inpatient speech-language pathology, Christina, on flute and another speech-language pathologist, Madeline, on violin—who selflessly donated their break times from their own sessions to play with us. Soon, we had a whole repertoire of songs for our newfound quartet! We practised and practised and the ensemble became more and more polished. The culmination of our efforts materialised in the form of a small 'concert', staged within the hospital's foyer. Libby's family, other patients and therapists in the hospital assembled to form the audience. This event held profound significance—the fact that she not only reached the point of delivering a thirty-minute concert but also mustered the endurance for it testified to her monumental progress. The concert became a time of celebration, uniting us in a shared appreciation for Libby's courageous spirit and the power of music therapy.

"When The Saints Go Marching In" was the closing number of the program's eight songs. It will always remain in my memory as a monumental milestone and accomplishment for Libby. This traditional spiritual song, a staple in American history that was famously recorded by Louis Armstrong & His Orchestra, also won't be forgotten in my career history.

Two months later, Libby's chapter at the hospital concluded as she was discharged, marking the continuation of her rehabilitation journey at home. Undeterred by the adversity that had unfolded for her and her family, she pursued her aspirations. She fulfilled her dream of attending college, graduating with a Bachelor of Science.

Her achievements extended even further across the globe as her studies led her to a prestigious university in the UK for a semester. These fantastic and impressive accomplishments, borne from her determined and positive outlook on life, are a testament to her capacity to transcend even the most difficult setbacks one could ever imagine. To have played a role in this journey is a privilege I hold dear and won't forget.

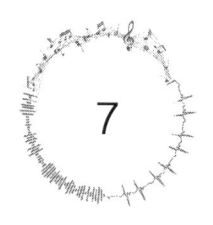

STAND TALL

Building resilience with children in adoption and foster care

"In the lap of music, we may discern unforeseen resilience."[70]
— Poet Rajbir Kaur

The United Nations has estimated that around 260,000 adoptions take place worldwide each year[71] and approximately 120 per 100,000 children are in foster or residential care.[72] Due to emotional adversity and trauma, children in care often get an unfair start to life and need extra support to increase their ability to develop resilience, self–esteem, concentration, regulation and sense of identity.

How music can help

Music therapy can be a powerful therapeutic tool to help children establish meaningful relationships and build self-esteem. Researcher Jo-Anne Lefevre states that "children rarely have the language or the cognitive development to process and convey their experiences solely through words, so more symbolic modes of communication and engagement have shown to be more successful when working directly with children."[73] Music therapists can use various elements in music-making and/or improvised music with language to help them externalise their emotions that can be unspeakable and confusing. Here, musical and verbal interactions can act as a containing function to help reduce patients' re-experiences of trauma or simply support their emotional lives.[74]

Music is also an inviting, playful and effective way to capture a child's attention, allowing the child to have a sense of control in their environment.[75] It provides a link between emotion and thought which can heighten the understanding of the expression of emotion,[76] enables them to find their voice and help them to express difficult feelings for the first time. Many children respond positively to music which encourages the experiences of positive emotions such as happiness, joy and security.[77]

A shared creative experience in music therapy can also allow the child a space to engage in positive play, giving them a chance to explore and build a new relationship. Research suggests activities that are structured, intended for building skills and require regular participation will produce positive effects, such as increasing self-esteem.[78] Furthermore, Varvara Pasiali, professor and researcher at Queens University of Charlotte, North Carolina, proposed that "music therapy as a playful and creative medium for children eventually becomes a powerful avenue to minimise the impact of stressful life circumstances".[79]

Meeting David

David was a participant in a research project that I undertook at an adoption and fostering agency, the concluding project of my master's degree. The project looked at ways in which music therapy might improve the self-esteem of adopted and fostered children, how it might help them face adversity and build resilience. He was eight years old at the time we started sessions and had been adopted at the age of two. At this point in his life, David was struggling to understand and accept his adoption and settle within his family. His low self-esteem struggles manifested into aggressive behaviour at home, which was becoming increasingly difficult for his adoptive mother to handle.

A special connection

The participating families in the project agreed to thirty-minute music therapy sessions for their child over eight weeks and an interview with the adoptive/foster parent upon conclusion of the sessions. Within the first few minutes of the first session, I knew that David had an incredible connection with music and he had a lot to say and process. Our sessions usually began with improvisation. I provided accompaniment on the keyboard or guitar and David would explore different instrumentation. Initially, he was always very sure of his actions musically but reluctant to speak. He was shy, choosing to play improvisations with no lyrics and explore the wide range of instruments on offer including drums, keyboard, guitar, metallophone, maracas and tambourines, rather than verbalise any words. During these improvisations, I worked to provide the resources and the creative environment to enable him to find his own path rather than being too directive within the sessions, allowing him to have a sense of control in his environment to create a permissive, child-centred atmosphere. The result was a lot of 'musical conversation', using solely instrumentation to communicate back and forth—we listened to each other, matched each other's rhythms and engaged in call-and-response dialogue. Client-therapist trust began to build.

The skill of improvising was a huge challenge and learning curve for me during my music therapy training. For twenty years prior I had solely read sheet music, however in the world of improvisation there are no little black dots on the page to refer back to. Luckily, David and I grew with confidence together and it became more natural and easier for me to follow his lead in the musical conversations.

Eventually, words began to flow. David was a big fan of musical theatre and during one improvisation he began singing about his feelings to the melody of "I Dreamed a Dream" from the Andrew Lloyd Webber musical Les Misérables. I was amazed when a strong and powerful singing voice emerged from such a small body!

> *I don't want to be treated anymore*
> *All I want is to be someone*
> *But why do I have to be treated and ignored*
> *All I do is get treated like garbage*
>
> *I feel not wanted anymore*
> *I only feel a company*
> *I want some help right now*
> *To be back in shape I could have an operation*
> *One that's going to make my feelings stay the same*

The purpose of the music therapist in building self-esteem and resilience revolves around nurturing and facilitating a child's journey towards self-awareness and a coherent sense of their place in the world. David was clearly questioning this, so at this point I intended to foster an environment where he felt empowered to navigate these introspective inquiries, encouraging him to have a safe space to express feelings while supporting him musically through thoughtful keyboard accompaniment and vocals.

He continued.

I feel like I'm a bit of a carrot, really good
But then you throw me away in the bin
But that's not how it feels sometimes in real life
But I just want to explode
You know like a can of Coke you fizz it up and well I just don't feel like that

During a weekly update with David's adoption support manager, I learned about a common belief felt by adopted children of being "no good because their parents gave them away because they were no good so they are going to prove them right." I was therefore becoming aware that any negative responses might lead him to feel devalued or a failure.

Fostering resilience within David's songwriting—standing tall

By this point, the outlook of the sessions shifted. David's adoption support manager and I agreed that it would be beneficial for him to focus on his good and positive feelings, 'standing tall' against his negative feelings towards himself. In our fifth session together we began an improvised song based on the title "Stand Tall". I implemented the idea for this after he sang the lyrics *I look like I'm getting older, but please make me stand tall* during an improvised song in the previous session. After speaking with his adoption support worker, we agreed that it would be beneficial for him to focus on his. I accompanied David on the keyboard, following his vocal melodies as he played the ocean drum—a circular drum with metal beads inside that imitates the sound of the ocean when tipped from side to side.

> *I'm sitting at my house*
> *Imagining there's a river*
> *Sailing round*
> *This place of nowhere*
>
> *I go right along*
> *Right up on my feet*
> *As I look*
> *I hear the music*
>
> *The river's getting deeper*
> *Going round*
> *We're going through a big storm*
> *Until we go to here*
>
> *Stand tall*
> *From the dangers*
> *That will erupt you*
> *From the dangers that will begin*

Musically, I supported him by matching the overall feeling of what he was singing and following his directions of when to stop and start within the song. I wanted him to hold the autonomy within the song and this composition served as a canvas for him to articulate his identity and emotions. Upon the conclusion of our sessions, this song was recorded and I presented David with a copy of the recording, encapsulating these transformative moments we shared.

During the post-session interview, David's mother reported a noteworthy transformation, sharing that "things have been better this summer than they were last summer". She observed a distinct shift in his behaviour, noting that "he is not as demonstrably angry as he was". She also highlighted that after each session he was "very happy when he came out" and noted a reduction in the frequency of his emotional outbursts, underscoring a positive stride in his emotional regulation.

A lasting personal effect

I was selected to present the research project at the American Music Therapy Association Passages Conference in upstate New York and the national conference in Louisville, Kentucky. It was an honour to share this work with other music therapists, fostering a sense of shared dedication to our field's advancement. My experiences from this research project remained with me long after graduation, serving as a guiding force and shaping my perspective.

Almost a decade later, the lasting influence of the research project and my time working with David and the other project participants remained, along with my passion to contribute meaningfully and substantially to the foster and adoptive community. This led me to embark on the journey of fostering myself. In October 2020, I passed the required interviews, training, checks and inspections to become a licensed foster parent in the State of North

Carolina. From that point onwards, I provided monthly respite weekend care for foster siblings for the remainder of my time there.

At the time of starting the research project, I had never found the courage to sing in public before. David's ultimate poise, fortitude and blossoming connection with his voice inspired me greatly. I began to sing backing vocals with local bands, eventually singing solo and in a duo. Vocal confidence is hugely important in music therapy work. Sessions are often led with the voice and in some instances, instruments are required to be removed completely from the therapy room if the client poses a threat to safety due to their behaviour.

The project also had a lasting effect on David. I was so happy to hear recently that he continued using his talents in musical theatre and acting groups throughout his teenage years and is now studying for a career in film.

8

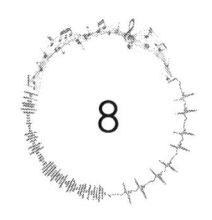

OH, WHAT A BEAUTIFUL MORNIN'

Reminiscing in dementia care

"The beautiful thing is, music can be like a time machine. One song—the lyrics, the melody, the mood—can take you back to a moment in time like nothing else can."[80]
- Writer Lisa Schroeder

Dementia is often called the cruellest of diseases because of the way it gradually strips people of their ability to function. At first, little things are brushed off as normal. It could be forgetting a few things, perhaps developing obsessive-compulsive disorder (OCD) tendencies. Then, the person can forget important details or something that has been explained multiple times, setting the stage for further challenges. Eventually, they likely may not be able to remember their loved ones or even their own name. A person with progressing dementia then feels confused more and more often. When they can't make sense of the world or if they get something wrong, they might feel frustrated or angry and annoyed with other people. They also may not even know they are upset and can't describe why they are experiencing these feelings.

Alzheimer's disease is the most common form of dementia, affecting one in nine people over sixty-five in the US[81] and one in fourteen in the UK.[82] When I began writing this chapter there were no known effective treatments to prevent, cure or slow the progression of the diseases that cause dementia. However, progress has been made. In July 2023 the US Food and Drug Administration (FDA) approved a medication thought to slow Alzheimer's[83], a massive breakthrough in dementia research and one which hopefully will herald a positive impact on countless lives in the future.

Music and memory

For someone with dementia who eventually may not be able to communicate, we know we can use songs to engage them. An overlap of musical memory regions has been observed with areas that are "relatively spared"[84] in Alzheimer's disease, thus explaining its surprising preservation even as other cognitive domains falter. This also explains why individuals with dementia often can't remember the names of their loved ones but can remember lyrics to songs from their teenage years. Despite losing much of their ability to communicate and with their short-term memory affected, music can connect individuals with dementia to what is meaningful for them and creates a sanctuary of solace and communion. As author and entrepreneur Michael Bassey Johnson states, "music replays the past memories, awakens our forgotten worlds and make our minds travel".[85]

Studies have shown music can even improve memory, with connectivity in the brain increasing.[86] A team of researchers at Northeastern University noticed that several pathways on both sides of the brain were activated by music, including the medial prefrontal cortex, which plays a significant regulatory role in decision-making and memory.[87] They also discovered that music bridged the gap between the brain's auditory system and reward system, the area that governs motivation. Researchers at the University of Utah also studied the brain's response to music listening in patients with a clinical diagnosis of Alzheimer's. Findings "supported a mechanism whereby attentional network activation in the brain's salience network may lead to improvements in brain network synchronisation"[88], anchoring hope in the potential of music to mitigate the afflictions of cognitive decline.

The need for more services

In 1991, thanks to the efforts of advocating music therapists led by Cathy Knoll, there was a transformative legislative stride in the United States. Senate bill S.1723, Music Therapy for Older Americans Act,[89] added music therapy to the lists of services for frail older individuals (particularly those with the greatest economic and social need) in their homes, designed to satisfy their particular needs and improve their quality of life. Music therapy was also added to lists of supportive services for schools within colleges and universities in which training programs in the field of ageing can be developed; services under the definition of 'preventive health services' and demonstration projects, which improve or expand supportive services or otherwise promote the well-being of older individuals. The legislative landscape has changed for the better due to this bill but unfortunately, I have seen many times that it often appears to be forgotten about within the budgets of memory care facilities. The struggle to find funding for much-needed music therapy services does not stop at memory care, however. In the United States, the sad reality is that only eleven states have licensure to make music therapy services reimbursable for health insurance companies and resources continue to diminish. According to recent research, advocacy burnout is one of the three main reasons that music therapists leave the profession.[90] Chapter 11 delves further into some of the difficulties of the profession.

The brain's response to music

Songs reminiscent of our early years can retrieve the memories and feelings of connection and safety we often feel in infancy and childhood. For seniors, this connection to music (whether experienced live or through recorded forms) resonates as an evocative bridge to bygone eras, echoing the words of essayist and writer Lance Morrow, that "music is the way our memories sing to us across time."[91] From a regulatory and therapeutic point of view, these songs have the capacity to instil a sense of control within our minds and allow our nervous system to feel safe.

It is also the movement of the simple melody in songs that make sense in a way that soothes the nervous system. Think of the repetitive melodies of "Edelweiss" and "Que Sera, Sera (Whatever Will Be, Will Be)" for example, where simplicity reigns and repetition works like magic. These compositions possess an intrinsic power to instil in our brains a reassuring sense of command over our surroundings, inducing a feeling of safety. It is repetition that creates a sense of predictability in our environment and leads our brain to think, "I know what's coming next!" When the same line, phrase or lyric repeats, our brain feels in control.

Often, the purpose of music therapy with the dementia population is to reconnect people with music. However, it is also important to note that older people may like the music of their generation, or they may not. Therefore, a music therapist must not make assumptions about what kind of music to use in a session when beginning to work with an older individual. Ultimately music preference is less important than client goals but there is a fine line with this—as previously noted in Chapter 6, acknowledging music preference often leads to increased client motivation.

Singing for the brain

Parkinson's disease is a neurological degenerative disease that often comes hand in hand with dementia. People with Parkinson's often have difficulty generating sequences and rhythms due to damage in a particular part of their brain called the substantia nigra which controls movement. They also often move too fast or move too slow. Music gives them back time, sequence, rhythm and a normal tempo.[92] There is also a gradual loss of dopamine producing neurons in the brain.

Professor Katherine Goforth Elverd has created a transformative initiative at The University of Tennessee, Chattanooga—an endeavour christened the 'Trembling Troubadours"[93]. This therapeutic choir serves as a haven for those navigating Parkinson's disease alongside their dedicated caregivers. Music can help with not only the motor movements impacted by Parkinson's in speaking but also breathing, vocal volume and articulation. The goal of the choir is exactly this—to increase breath support, vocal intensity and articulation, offering a lifeline to dimensions afflicted by the disease's grip. Each rehearsal starts with physical and vocal warm-ups, leading into rehearsing well-known and loved songs that reverberate across generations.

I also recently read about a community choral group in Minnesota for people aged 55 plus,[94] with the oldest member being an astounding 99 years old. The choir memorises their whole concert of music spanning the centuries from the 1800s to The Beatles.

The testimonies of Victoria Butler and Marylee Fithian[95], members of each respective choir, encapsulate the ineffable essence of their shared journeys:

"It has been a major help for me in my struggle with coping with the symptoms of Parkinson's Disease...it has helped me add structure to my days and I no longer feel a need to

be invisible because of PD. I also feel like by participating, I help myself and I contribute to the wellbeing of others with this challenge."

"It keeps our brains active and fills our lives in ways that nothing else can. I don't think that at this stage in my life, anything makes me happier. And just as important is the joy it brings to our audience as they listen and sing along."

The benefits of group singing are noticed all over the world. A recent study of neurological and community choirs in New Zealand reported several benefits associated with choral singing, identified under psychological, social relationships and environmental domains.[96]

Stimulating senses

Anxiety and depression are common in nursing homes as individuals often feel they can no longer make choices for themselves and may struggle with the perceived loss of autonomy and independence. Music therapy helps maintain social and verbal skills, stimulates recall and increases cognition. It allows them to maintain or build self-esteem, building a community to empower them to speak up, articulate opinions and make choices. Music can also help older adults socialise and decrease isolation. It serves as a catalyst for dialogue and stimulates discussions rich with shared memories. However, as mentioned in Chapter 3, music therapy may also pave a pathway for distressing recollections to reappear. An essential part of a music therapist's work is to help the patient process the memories that may surface. Otherwise, this can be upsetting for them—especially if the memories include loved ones who have passed away or other difficult memories. Care and consideration must be taken when preparing other music modalities such as personalised playlists of recorded music for this reason.

Music therapy gives a shared experience, a connection and human contact formed while being part of a music experience. All these things can hugely impact mood and, ultimately, quality of life, also likely leading to better compliance with the health care provided to them. And, of course, it gives an opportunity to work on physical range of motion and movement through instrumental playing, stretching and dancing.

It is also important to note that while music therapy is a multi-sensory activity, finding the balance between stimulation and calming is paramount. Some individuals thrive amidst vibrant sensory landscapes that ignite their engagement and spark connections. For them, the rhythm and cadence of music serve as catalysts, propelling them into a state of heightened engagement. Some may feel distressed with too many jumbled and confused thoughts, so music can help to break through the chaos of their mind in ways that nothing else can. Others, however, find solace in the tranquillity that music can offer—its soothing cadences and gentle melodies provide a refuge and an oasis of calm. Therefore, the challenge for the music therapist in memory care groups, or essentially any music therapy group, is to orchestrate an experience that simultaneously nurtures both stimulation and tranquillity, treading the fine line between engagement and comfort. The therapeutic skill lies in underpinning the music, producing an environment that respects and accommodates these variations for each individual and fostering an inclusive space where everyone is involved and every sensory threshold is acknowledged.

On top of all this, some people just 'go for it!' with instruments and singing, others need much more encouragement. It's a balance of attunement, sensitivity and adaptability, creating an atmosphere that ensures each participant finds resonance, regardless of their unique sensory landscape.

I was lucky to have experienced first-hand all of the above early in my music therapy career. After graduating in 2013 in the UK, I volunteered at a memory care facility in Pitlochry, Scotland. I then moved to the US at the end of the year and requirements for board certification from the Certification Board for Music Therapists meant I had to undertake two additional internships. I was very fortunate to find music therapist Melissa Simmons, who kindly volunteered her time to supervise me at a hospice and memory care facility in Florida, where I witnessed the special connections she created with clients. This was also where I quickly realised that I had decades of American folk and traditional music to learn! My first true realisation of how much repertoire music therapists need to know and have prepared in their 'toolbox' for any situation—the answer is a LOT!

Camille and her new lease on life

Shortly after finishing my internships, I moved to New Jersey and began a contract at a senior living facility which included a memory care wing. A few weeks after starting the contract, I met Camille. Camille was approaching her ninetieth birthday and this was her first week participating in the group music therapy sessions. I noticed Camille first in the group because she was not participating; her shoulders slumped in her chair with her head down. She looked as if she had given up on life. While meeting with her care workers, I was informed that she had recently arrived at the care home and hated everything about it.

A few minutes into the session I began the song "Oh, What a Beautiful Mornin'", the opening song from the Broadway musical *Oklahoma*. After the first line of the chorus, she sat upright and lifted her head, her posture radiating renewed energy and vitality. Her face lit up and she began to sing every word until the end of the song while tapping her feet. Witnessing Camille embrace the music with her voice and feet was such a surprise and a moment I will never forget.

Her daughter stopped me in the hall the following week. She had tears in her eyes. It turned out that "Oh, What a Beautiful Mornin'" was a song her father sang to her as a child. He had sadly passed away a few years earlier. This song brought back so many happy memories for Camille, transporting her to happy times and resurrecting a cherished bond that stretched across the ages. It instantly transformed her whole being. This song will always remind me of Camille—the instant transformation it brought and her new lease of life.

Camille remained a lively member of the group and I also facilitated weekly individual sessions with her, encouraging her to be more comfortable in her environment by emphasizing sensory awareness using different auditory and tactile stimulation including the rain stick, scarves and the lap harp.

Working with Camille early in my career brought me so much joy. I then went on to lead many more groups in memory care facilities in New Jersey and North Carolina and I was lucky to create many more memories like this in the following years.

9

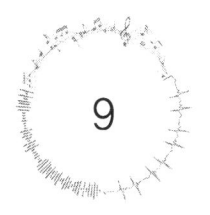

PAIN DON'T HURT ME NO MORE

Encouraging self-expression through songwriting

"Songwriting is a great release. It helps me work through things."[97]

- Musician Jo Dee Messina

You will have already seen many examples of moving and memorable songwriting in the previous chapters. It may look simple to some, but in reality, many people are intimidated by the term songwriting. "I could never write a song!" is a phrase I have often heard. Fortunately, there are ways to make songwriting accessible and inviting within music therapy, especially for those who haven't tried it before. One such approach is 'piggybacking' (sometimes referred to as 'mad libs'), a creative technique of taking pre-composed songs with a familiar tune and creating a new set of lyrics. You may remember David in Chapter 7 who unknowingly improvised a piggy-backing song to the tune of "I Dreamed a Dream" from the musical *Les Misérables.*

Piggybacking is an effective way to introduce songwriting because it gives structure and a template to work with and the music therapist can help guide the process. After beginning with piggybacking song exercises, I have seen many budding songwriters build confidence and then go on to create original compositions from scratch in sessions. At this stage, the music therapist's role can also evolve, subsequently helping to compose and set the music along with the lyrics. Piggybacking has been so beneficial in my work across many different populations and settings with a wide range of conditions, from detox substance abuse units and day programs for developmental disabilities to oncology wards and behavioural health units. Some examples of previous piggybacking exercises are shown below.

1. To encourage sharing feelings, I used the tune of James Brown's song "I Got You (I Feel Good)". This songwriting excerpt was from a session I facilitated with a patient diagnosed with global developmental delay. An individual with this condition is delayed in all areas of development, presenting challenges in understanding emotions and feelings, social interactions, self-expression and daily functioning.

> *I'm a bit sad*
> *When people aren't nice to each other*
> *I'm a bit sad*
> *When people aren't nice to each other*
> *A bit sad, A bit sad*
> *When people aren't nice to each other*

> *I am proud*
> *When I take care of my emotions*
> *I am proud*
> *When I take care of my emotions*
> *I'm proud, I'm proud*
> *When I take care of my emotions*

After the patient wrote these lyrics, we discussed them, during which I offered validation for her emotions. I encouraged her to delve deeper into why she felt this way, providing examples and prompts when required. Many times I have seen patients, who had never shared anything before this songwriting moment, sharing and sometimes even recognising their emotions for the first time during this exercise. Sitting with the patient while they process these feelings and empathising with them is therefore a big part of the therapeutic process in this context.

2. To encourage patients to reflect on their own world and think about what is positive and meaningful in their lives, I used the tune of the well-known song "What a Wonderful World" by Louis Armstrong. This example was taken from an inpatient substance abuse detox group.

> *The flowers are so bright*
> *In the garden outside*
> *The scent so sweet, the colors are neat*
> *And I think to myself...*
>
> *I think of my family*
> *Caring about me*
> *Soon they'll be near, when I leave here*
> *And I think to myself...*

The above example has been one of my favourite piggy-backing songwriting exercises over the years due to its versatility. Over time, I have had the privilege of hearing so many different versions at different life stages. One of the things I love the most about my work in music therapy is constantly being surprised about how creative people can be (and that creativity is often suppressed) and how one short and simple excerpt of a song can unearth such deep inner feelings, memories and reflections.

3. To increase comfort for a patient in the hospital, I used the tune of the Woody Guthrie song "This Land is Your Land" to create the song "These Are the Things that Make Me Me". During this exercise, I encourage the patient to talk about their favourite things and maybe some things they don't like to create an atmosphere of familiarity and ease. This example was taken from a session with a paediatric patient in an epilepsy monitoring unit (EMU). As mentioned in the Introduction, the EMU requires children to be affixed to a monitor via a network of wires glued to their heads, a requirement that spans twenty-four hours or more. This duration can pose a significant test to the patience of younger patients and, at times, evoke apprehension and fear.

My name is Avery
And I like music
Playing with my sisters
And dancing at school
I love macaroni and cheese
But I don't like medicines
These are the things that make me me

4. I used the tune of the song "This is Me" from the biographical musical drama film *The Greatest Showman* to empower and develop resilience. This example is from a session with a patient struggling with depression and suicidal ideations.

> *My name is Valentina*
> *And I like to roar*
> *I feel strong and powerful*
> *I am not a stranger here today*
> *I am victorious*
> *I am a champion*
>
> *They will not say mean things to me*
> *Because there is a place for me*
> *I am a warrior*

After completing this exercise, I prompted the patient to articulate her feelings, reflecting post-session. Her written response reads as follows:

"I think the songwriting has made me more musical and more understanding. And I feel accepted and safe."

Davina sings her story

Davina's story unfolds through a series of excerpts from her songs, selected from a collection of many, many more. Davina was twenty-four when I worked with her and, at the time, was diagnosed with oppositional defiant disorder (ODD) and intermittent explosive disorder—a mental health disorder characterised by frequent impulsive anger outbursts or aggression. Her mother had spent most of her life in and out of jail, a background that had inevitably influenced Davina's life. This upbringing, combined with years spent navigating through group homes and transitional housing, led to her journey being entrapped in a relentless cycle. She desperately needed an outlet for expression.

Before the first session, the behavioural health technicians on the unit had informed me that she was a huge fan of hip-hop and rap music. What no one was aware of at the time, however, was her extraordinary gift for freestyling rap. I soon found this out around five minutes into the first session.

I would join her in the initial stages by improvising on the keyboard to complement her vocals, although it quickly became apparent that the raps demanded a stronger and more supportive beat. Using GarageBand, the Apple music software writing program mentioned previously in Chapter 5, I guided her through the process of creating a series of different backing tracks that could provide the necessary support for her lyrical expressions. She used pre-composed loops, dedicating considerable time and precision to layer and arrange them to create her desired sounds. When she was happy with the finished product, the beat started, the words soon flowed and didn't stop flowing often for ten minutes straight.

Davina had an instant and deep connection with music, rising to her feet in the room as soon as the beat started, embracing the sounds with closed eyes.

In the first session, she began with an expression of reflection and self-exploration:

"Feelings Song"

I woke up this morning
Feeling kind of meh, but ready for the day
Thinking about me, feeling so wild and free
Feeling the unknown

Subsequently, she continued along the path of introspection interlaced with moments of poignant sorrow. Her continued narrative explored the subject of the termination of her relationship with her mother.

"Never Forget"

I'll never forget those moments that we had
You're with me forever, you're by my side
Yes, you and me
I'll never forget the times that we had

Davina's journey then shifted towards a phase of contemplation and reflection. Her lyrics delved into embracing emotions of pain, anger, confusion and bewilderment.

"How I Feel"

Cause I'm hurting
Hurting like the storm
Like the rain it's coming
The storm and the rain are causing all the pain

People say that I'm not any different from you
People they don't know how I feel
They used to call me this and then they used to call me that
Oh no, I refuse to let you go

This evolution led her to a place of self-acceptance, where a newfound confidence also began to form.

"Pain Don't Hurt Me No More"

That everybody she sees cares about her
She says, she says she's lonely
I hope that she knows she's loved
I hope that she feels like she can be free

Every day I see her
I'll tell you something now
They care about me
Pain don't hurt me no more

"Pain Don't Hurt Me No More" was memorable because I noticed a shift in Davina's positivity after this song. Subsequently, her lyrical themes began to weave narratives of hope and aspirations for the future.

"Hopes and Dreams"

She had a dream that one day
You will see her walk across the stage
Now I'm singing this song
One day these hopes and dreams will happen

Everyone's there with me, everybody starts to dance
It's time to celebrate, it's gonna be great
It's time to live my life
Everybody sing, sing this song with me

"Future"

She can reach and grab it
That's all I wanna do
All this time I've been living in this world
Can't take it with me

Every day I'm thinking
'Bout this future, 'bout the stars
My future it shines so bright
She's one step closer to her future

What I found interesting, along with her exceptional talent, was that Davina never had one aggressive outburst throughout our sessions, which often spanned over an hour. Evidently, the space cultivated by her music therapy sessions provided her with a safe and non-threatening space for her self-expression to thrive. That we had managed to maintain this progress while working together for so long was a testament to our collaboration and an achievement that resonated deeply with me.

Calvin's story

Calvin's tumultuous upbringing was evident when I first met him. Aged seventeen, he had spent much of his life moving between group homes and behavioural health units and bore the heavy weight of a challenging childhood. As a result of the absence of parental support and guidance, he was hugely lacking in self-assurance and a clear sense of his life's trajectory. Despite this, Calvin's character shone with an undeniable charisma, a sharp wit and a playful grin. He was curious, open-minded and observant of the world and people around him.

Calvin was very interested in the guitar, primarily due to the fond memories he held of his father playing when he was a child. Beyond its sentimental significance, the guitar offered him a tangible outlet to channel his energies and focus, particularly during extended stays in the behavioural health unit caused by delays in the state care system. I introduced Calvin to a few guitar chords, which he picked up immediately, beginning to strum between E minor and A minor. This alternating chord progression creates a somewhat moody and reflective sound and the repetition and simplicity leave room for compelling lyrics. It wasn't long before these started in the form of spoken word.

> *Remember where you're from*
> *For the war is never won*
> *Because I am a son of a son*
> *And the world has just begun*
> *For things in life are not fun*
> *Stay in school for the bell has rung*
>
> *As I'm writing this song*
> *Some places I just don't belong*
> *Some things I achieved*
> *All I had to do was believe*
> *I wonder what life will be like for me*
> *But right now I feel like everything is make-believe*
>
> *Don't reminisce*
> *There's things you'll never forget*
> *For life I will be set*
> *Just never regret*
> *But I think that's all I got to say*
> *Till another day*
> *I hope anyway*
>
> *My life is starting to fade*
> *But that's all the facts I can say*
> *Just know I'm going the other way*
> *What do you say?*

A progression from past reflections blossoming into a celebration of confidence and self-worth was noted as Calvin expressed that he wanted to transition from spoken word to song, so I helped him to set melodies to his words. This transformation was poignantly encapsulated in the chorus of his song "This is My Life".

The past is gone
The future is now
Just like a king come up and receive your crown
A little bit older now
And I'm in a small town
Thinking about how I'll look up not down
This is my life

Finally, an ending of self-acceptance and a promising outlook for the future is epitomised in the chorus of his song "The Right Path".

I'm on the right path now
As good as I can see
I'm on the right path now
This is the right place to be
So I'll just focus on me, focus on me

As shown in this chapter and throughout the book, songwriting is a powerful vehicle for storytelling and expression. It was an immense privilege to play a role in the evocative narratives both Davina and Calvin told. Bearing witness to their profound journeys of self-discovery and growth was truly inspirational.

10

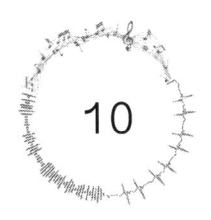

NO ONE LIKE YOU

Commemorating music for new beginnings and the end of life

"Music is an important part of our physical and emotional well-being, ever since we were babies in our mother's womb listening to her heartbeat and breathing rhythms."[98]
- Clinical psychologist Franz Wendtner

Music therapists work with individuals from birth to the end of life. These two moments are universal to all living beings and in my opinion, from what I have seen and experienced, it is pertinent for both of these times in life to be dignified and poignant—especially if there are unforeseen difficulties or complications.

The first few years of life have been extensively documented as the most important developmentally for an infant. In fact, during this time, according to research at the University of Harvard, more than one million neural connections are formed every second.[99] It has been proven that children who learn to make music early in life have advantages, particularly in language development.[100] Music's influence can promote prosocial behaviour,[101] mediate fast social bonding,[102] and increase trust and cooperation.[103] In fact, studies have shown that practising music at an early age can also make structural changes to the brain that stay with you for the rest of your life.[104]

When caregivers sing to their infants, they intuitively support the caregiver-infant social bond and social learning, simultaneously increasing the infant's language exposure. What is equally fascinating are two research findings: children a year after they were born recognizing and preferring music they had been exposed to in the womb,[105] and the ability of infants as young as five months to distinguish between happy and sad musical excerpts.[106] Music therapists have also supported mothers with their physical and emotional needs, effectively utilising music to calm, block discomfort and direct focus on breathing during labour and childbirth. This has been shown to decrease anxiety and the need for analgesic medications significantly during birth, ultimately contributing to overall positive feelings about the birth process.[107]

The opposite side of the spectrum—the end of life—is an emotionally charged and heartbreaking time. There is often fear and dread, not only for the patient but also for their loved ones who are beginning the grieving period as they see the patient go through the end-of-life process. It is commonly a time of reflection and reminiscence, which music can support effectively. There have been many instances in hospital and hospice work where I was able to be there with patients during their final moments, providing comfort and solace through playing their favourite music. This often encompassed tunes that held meaning throughout their lives or spiritual melodies that resonated with their religious beliefs. Matching the patient's breath with the tempo of the music and gradually slowing down the tempo to calm the mind and body can also gently guide the patient's state of mind and body, creating a calming effect and sense of tranquillity. Playlists moving from faster songs (100-120 bpm) to slower songs (60- 80 bpm) can also cue a relaxation response. A few years ago, I also helped a patient to write a song dedicated to all the people in her life who were meaningful to her.

The smallest patients

During the years I worked in children's hospitals, I spent a lot of time working with the smallest of patients in the Neonatal Intensive Care Unit (NICU) and their families, using music to soothe crying infants with live lullabies and a vertical rocking technique alongside a repertoire of acapella melodies to calm and induce sleep. This work was hard as it is intensive and worrisome working with the most fragile of patients. It is also surprisingly tiring to sing a cappella at a low volume for long periods of time.

Instrumentation can also be used to promote developmental stimulation for NICU babies, including mimicking the sounds of the mother's womb using an ocean disc[108] and playing a low-pitched drum that emulates a heartbeat (as mentioned in the Introduction) to comfort and soothe the infant. Great care was always taken in the NICU so that the output decibel level remained attuned to the developmental thresholds of each individual infant.

Sometimes, an infant unfortunately does not have the best start in life. One such instance is a diagnosis of Neonatal Abstinence Syndrome (NAS), a group of conditions stemming from the infant's withdrawal from opioids or other harmful drugs they were exposed to in utero from their mother's drug use while pregnant. This complex array of conditions encompasses tremors, seizures, twitching, tight muscle tone, persistent high-pitched crying, respiratory difficulties, disrupted sleep patterns, poor feeding and slow weight gain. The gravity of poor feeding and slow weight gain cannot be overstated, as adequate infant nutrition is essential for growth, well-being and overall development. Poor nutrition increases the risk of illness and can also lead to obesity—a pressing public health problem in many countries.[109]

For NAS patients (and other premature infants with poor feeding for varying reasons), a piece of technology to promote feeding was developed by Florida State University: the Pacifier Activated Lullaby (PAL). This innovative machine consists of a sensor attached to a pacifier, which is then connected to a speaker system housing pre-recorded acapella lullabies. When the infant latches on to the pacifier and produces an effective suck to activate the player, the speaker plays music as a 'reward'. Seeing infants as young as a few hours old 'catch on' to this was truly incredible. The lullabies on the speaker are specifically selected for their simple three-chord structure and have minimal large intervals from one note to the next, minimising the risk of overstimulation for the infant. The sensor level required to activate the speaker can also be increased. By augmenting the effort required for an infant to trigger the musical response, the infant is trained to produce a more efficient suck from the bottle. As a result, these infants transition to feeding sooner and tolerate feedings better. Studies have shown that the use of the PAL. reduces hospital stay time for premature and NAS infants by an average of five days.[110]

A new patent-pending invention, LullaFeed, created by board-certified Michael Detmer and infant feeding specialist and speech-language pathologist Rebekah Gossom, is a music-based, research-backed feeding device that attaches to virtually any baby bottle. LullaFeed plays music upon detecting when the baby is drinking, helping parents and feeding specialists support babies through the feeding progression with music.[111]

Liliana's NICU journey

Liliana was only three months old when I first met her and was already battling a recent genetic lung condition diagnosis. She had been a patient in the NICU since birth and was required to remain in the incubator until she could breathe independently. This consequently compromised the newborn bonding time and skin-to-skin contact with her parents. As a result, in the beginning, one of her music therapy goals was to increase parent-infant bonding and socialisation.

I remember the first time I arrived at the bedspace to introduce myself and music therapy services to Liliana's parents. The atmosphere was quiet and solemn. Their faces bore the weight of concern, visibly tired after months spent in the hospital, facing the unknown. Yet, the instant our dialogue shifted to the topic of Liliana, their faces lit up. She was their first-born child and was a bright light amid the uncertainties that had enveloped their lives.

I chose to piggyback a song, a technique elaborated upon in the previous chapter, using the melody of the beautiful John Denver song "No One Like You". I engaged in collaborative sessions with Lilliana's parents, prompting them to share details about their cherished daughter, encompassing her physical attributes, distinctive traits and her blossoming personality.

With their insights as my guide, I selected and rearranged what they loved the most and added them to the song. An excerpt of the song is shown below.

> *I love your smile*
> *I love your little nose*
> *I love your snuggles*
> *Your fingers and your toes*
>
> *You are a fighter*
> *Our little angel*
> *We can't wait to hug you*

Both parents appreciated this time and loved the song. Even Dad joined in on the singing! Liliana clearly did, too. She consistently sustained her gaze, locking eyes with her parents and smiling whenever they were singing. Music therapy was something Liliana's parents said they looked forward to during their long and demanding days on the unit. I also loved seeing her parents' eyes light up when talking about their daughter and giving them this experience to bond with her, even with the physical limitations.

A few weeks later, Liliana was ready for discharge. Her care continued at home and her condition was fortunately able to be medically managed so she could live a full and active life. She is now a thriving toddler, embodying the strength exemplified throughout her story. The verses of the song remain framed in her bedroom as a reminder of the first tough but resilient chapter of her life.

The heart beats on

Heartbeats signify life. Our bodies are musical—our steps follow a rhythm, our breathing flows to a tempo and our heart beats with a distinct rhythm of its own.

For some patients, life sadly ends too soon. In such poignant circumstances, music therapists can also extend their compassionate care to create something tangible for the family to keep as a lasting memory of their loved one, offered as a process within the context of the music therapy relationship. One such intervention is the heartbeat recording technology pioneered by music therapist Brian Schreck in 2014 during his time at Cincinnati Children's Hospital. Brian had the idea of connecting a digital stethoscope to *GarageBand* software to capture a live recording of the patient's heartbeat.[112] The result is now what is known as ACPR—amplified cardiopulmonary recordings. ACPR is an incredible piece of technology with the recorded heartbeat having remarkable clarity. As Brian expressively articulates in an episode of the *Enhance Life with Music* podcast;

> *"The body itself, as a symphony of life, can be used to create music."*[113]

Families can then choose what to record or loop over the top of the heartbeat, embellishing it with additional layers of significance. It is a collaborative process with as much input from the patient and/or family as possible. ACPR has been used during many different end-of-life circumstances, from traumatic accidents and hospice care to perinatal palliative care for infants who have been diagnosed with a terminal or life-limiting illness.[114]

Thanks to the generous support of a foundation grant, we were fortunate also to have the opportunity to bring the heartbeat recording to our hospital during my time there. Some families chose to record the heartbeat individually, some decided to have a song recorded over the beat that the family and music therapist had created or a version of the patient's favourite song. For the youngest patients, a soothing melody such as "Twinkle, Twinkle, Little Star" or another well-known public domain lullaby was often the most comforting for the family. Some hospitals also offer placing the heartbeat recording inside stuffed animals, providing additional comfort for the family, especially for siblings.

Facilitating this for families has been in equal parts emotional, draining and rewarding for me. Emotions are multi-faceted during this process—from the deep empathy required to underpin each interaction to the drain on one's emotional reserves. However, the intrinsic reward, the knowledge of having bestowed families with a treasure that encapsulates their bond with their loved ones, renders every endeavour unequivocally worthwhile. I am grateful to have provided this memory for many families to cherish.

Commemorating Cole's new life chapter

The heartbeat recording technology can also be used for heart transplant patients. A heart transplant also comes hand in hand with many emotions—excitement, relief, fear, the unknown of how the operation will go and whether the body will accept or reject the new heart. The heartbeat is recorded before and after the transplant, so this momentous chapter of life and a new beginning for the patient is permanently commemorated.

Cole, a twelve-year-old patient at Levine Children's Hospital who underwent a heart transplant, described the significance of his keepsake recorded by my co-worker Danae, another member of the music therapy team.

> *"To hear the difference is really cool. How I could hear my old and new heart was amazing."*[115]

Cole's mother echoed this, expressing that

> *"being able to know and keep where we've come from, we will take with us forever."*[116]

The heartbeat recording becomes a sonic bridge between past and present, a living testament to courage and transformation.

Music therapy treating the whole person

This chapter has shed light on interventions that embrace the spectrum of life's beginnings and ends. However, all times of life are just as meaningful in music therapy work. As articulated by Nurse Practitioner Lisa Lam at Levine Children's Hospital in Charlotte, North Carolina:

"We are not just here to fix a broken bone or surgically repair a heart; we are here to make sure that the patient and the family are cared for physically, mentally, emotionally and spiritually."[117]

To me, this perfectly encapsulates the true essence and importance of music therapy. Being a music therapist is more than just a job. It is about the care, empathy and connection towards each individual in need and the compassion felt when helping others. I hope this book has reflected that.

While writing this book I have constantly been reminded of the beauty that underscores the work of music therapists. It is in the gentle sounds that comfort an infant, the harmonies that bridge generations and the melodies accompanying each journey. It is in the shared songs that echo through hospital corridors and the compositions that etch memories into the heart, a reminder that healing is not confined to prescriptions and procedures; it encompasses the full spectrum of the human experience. Through the power of music therapy, we honour life in its entirety and in doing so, it stands as a testament to the depth of expression and the boundless capacity of empathy.

11

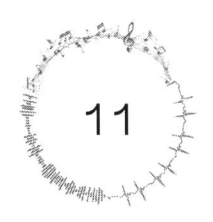

SOMEWHERE OVER THE (OTHER SIDE OF THE) RAINBOW

Reflecting on some of the challenges of the profession

"And when it rains on your parade, look up rather than down. Without the rain, there would be no rainbow."[118]
- Writer and Philosopher Gilbert K. Chesterton

As music therapist Judy Belland reflects in her informative and honest article[119] in the *Music Therapy Clinician* about the realities of a career in music therapy, I also want to be careful not to sugarcoat the reality of the field. Being a music therapist is not an easy job for many reasons. I have had sessions that have been less successful than the ones mentioned in this book including instruments being thrown across the room, aggressive verbal and physical outbursts, elopements leading to running across car parks, the requirement of physical restraints, a lot of screaming and too many bodily fluids to remember. Music therapist Roia Rofieyan in her reflective article[120] also shares the difficulty with clients who often do unexpected things—as a result you may be on edge for long periods of time while dealing with uncomfortable feelings. Therapists also need to watch for any contraindications (factors making the therapy inadvisable because it may be harmful) or if there is anything detrimental that happens while working with a client, for example a client having a seizure, which would require the session to be stopped. Both these instances can be stressful.

Human behaviour is complex, so naturally music therapy is also complex. Physical and emotional boundaries with clients have to be maintained even when some clients thrive on pushing the boundaries with their therapists. There have been times when I have had to navigate transference (the client's emotional reaction to the therapist) and countertransference (the therapist's emotional reaction to the client). Families have questioned their loved one's progress or change, unaware that each individual therapy journey progresses at very different rates. There have been sessions where I have had doubts about my abilities and times where a patient has regressed so I have worried that they aren't benefiting from the sessions. These are natural and common feelings to have considering how much skill and knowledge music therapists need to accumulate with all the different populations served, on top of being multi-instrumentalists, knowing a plethora of musical styles, genres and accompaniments.

As well as these difficulties, the physical location of the work can also be problematic. Institutions where many music therapists work can be noisy and ugly and from my experience music therapists frequently face challenges in securing adequate workspace—often relegated to the smallest available area, if we get a space at all. A huge hospital where I worked assigned us a cupboard with no windows as an 'office' for a team of two therapists and a university intern for the four years I was there. I remember one memory care facility where I was told to facilitate a session in a huge, open and busy day area (completely inappropriate for therapy) and halfway through the session a staff member in the kitchen directly behind me began crushing ice to make slushies for the residents. The noise was so loud I was unable to hear myself. There were also countless times I had a session scheduled with patients in different locations, only to turn up and someone else was using the room.

I would say that more often than not, music therapy is poorly understood and usually undervalued and we are constantly having to advocate for ourselves that we work an actual profession. I have encountered many staff, family members of patients I've worked with and even co-workers who haven't taken me or the field seriously. Some have even shown resentment that my job is 'easy' or have thought of music therapy as solely a distraction for the patients if they had nothing better to do. Some staff thought nothing of interrupting sessions or causing patients to miss their music therapy session completely. On top of this, I have seen insurance companies slash coverage of services with absolutely no advance warning to therapists or families—incredibly disheartening to say the least.

I have experienced burnout and compassion fatigue from the emotional toll and demanding environments, especially during the pandemic. I have also had to make many sacrifices in my personal life to allow me to continue being a music therapist. The inconsistent nature of contract work can be very stressful and low salaries with healthcare conglomerates (even with a master's degree) take a toll on financial health. If you decide to open a private practice, you are building a business in an "ever-growing commercial world".[121] On one hand, there's a desire to avoid overly commercialising a field rooted in compassion and kindness, while on the other, there's the practical necessity of having to make a living. It's a challenging path that involves balancing both ethical considerations—including client privacy if marketing online or on social media—and the realities of financial sustainability.

These reasons contribute to the growing number of music therapists leaving the field and music therapy students switching to other degree programmes. According to recent research published in the journal *Voices: A World Forum for Music Therapy,* the top three reasons for qualified therapists leaving the profession are availability of sustainable jobs, access to professional support or supervision and burden of advocacy.[122]

Despite all of these challenges and difficulties, I know that the moments I have described in each chapter, and many more like it, have made a career in music therapy so worthwhile.

12

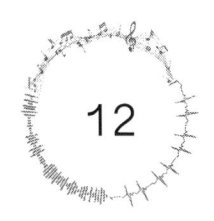

A NOTE TO THE TRAINEE MUSIC THERAPIST

Giving some helpful tips and advice to trainee music therapists and anyone considering a career in music therapy

"Let the beauty of what you love be what you do."[123]
- 13th-century poet Rumi

These thoughts are only my own and result from personal experience (and many hard lessons learned!). First, don't put too much pressure on yourself while training to be a music therapist! Don't forget that we need to be therapists, composers, performers and listeners simultaneously all the time. A tremendous amount of information and skills are required to complete a music therapy degree program, including proficiency in playing multiple instruments. In addition, we must think on our feet, be intuitive and empathic and adapt to the moment. We encounter difficult situations, heavy emotions and complex behaviours. As music therapists, we are wearing a lot of hats and spinning a lot of plates at the same time. During a single session, we might be doing all of the following:

- Playing the music, including using various meters and rhythms for accompaniment
- Adjusting the music in the moment to meet the client's needs
- Transposing the key of a song in the moment if necessary
- Observing the client's physical or emotional responses to the music
- Collecting data for goals the client(s) are working towards
- Asking questions to support the client's growth and awareness
- Talking with the client about the music therapy process
- Keeping note of music and musical experiences that the client(s) connects with
- Maintaining boundaries with the client(s)
- Cleaning the instruments after each session
- Reporting to the caregiver or family post-session with progress updates

We also do all of this while giving 100% in every session, which requires endless continual energy. It is easy to forget this and get burned out when you give so much and are not 'refilling your cup'. A little bit of advice:

- Make connections who will support you and understand you
- Take time to enjoy music for you!

- Avoid making music too 'clinical'—this is a fine line and problem for many artists whose passion becomes a job. For music therapists, *clinification*[124] happens when music becomes more clinical and less personally enjoyable, which causes personal music engagement to be neglected or stopped. Clinification can be concerning because your connection to music is essential. A disconnection with music can lead to burnout, being disconnected from something you love or losing touch with why you became a music therapist.

- Remember that being a music therapist is a lifelong learning process! Given the huge scope of music therapy practice encompassing so many different populations, it is simply impossible to learn and know everything after graduating. And that's okay! The most important thing is remaining receptive and willing to continue learning and expanding your knowledge and skills.

Music therapy job availability can also be limited. Unfortunately they, and arts positions in general, are always the ones to be withdrawn first when there are budget cuts. This is likely because most music therapy positions (especially in the United States) do not make the company money and many are only reimbursable by insurance companies if they are located in states with music therapy licensure. Furthermore, in the United States the sad reality is that many jobs only have benefits or health insurance if they are full-time. In this case, you may be better off finding another part-time job with benefits and 'topping up' your hours with music therapy work.

As I mentioned in the Introduction, when I first started my career in music therapy, I began with a hospital contract of only four hours a week while working three other non-music therapy jobs. Don't put pressure on yourself to get a full-time job right away—sometimes it's good to build up to a full-time caseload or even never have a full-time caseload if you feel it is too much. Only you know how much you can put 100% into and the hours will likely soon build up—in my case, up to twenty-four hours within my first year.

A music therapist's output is often far greater than the input, so it is imperative also to find the time for self-care and to recharge. Supervision is required and often individual counselling is needed too. I loved my time supervising and teaching undergraduate music therapy students—don't forget to reach out if you have questions!

Lastly, never forget the reasons why you decided to become a music therapist! It is the moments like I have described in this book that make the job and career worth it. These moments are priceless and the memories can never be taken away or replaced with any monetary value.

CONCLUDING THOUGHTS

As you will know by now after reading this book, I have been very fortunate to have spent much of my career thus far working with many different populations and age groups. However, there are still more populations served by music therapists that I have not mentioned. A few examples include music therapists who work in hundreds of correctional facilities and prisons around the world, some work with victims of human trafficking and children of domestic abuse victims, with refugees, minimally conscious patients, visually impaired and hard-of-hearing individuals. It is my opinion that for anyone in need of help in their lives, I am almost certain that music therapy will be able to benefit them in some way.

It is also important to note that for some people music therapy may not be the right therapy for them so an assessment must be undertaken before creating a treatment plan. Many different types of assessment tools and scales are used in music therapy; some are listed in the References section for those interested in learning more. For carers who are considering this type of therapy for your loved ones, or for anyone considering it for themselves, the best thing to do is to try it out and see if it works for them or for you.

I also wanted to reiterate that my approach to my music therapy practice is a culmination of my master's training program, coupled with my subsequent experience and additional certifications and training over the years. There are, in fact, many different approaches to music therapy including behavioural, developmental, neurologic, Nordoff-Robbins improvisational, psychodynamic and psychotherapeutic. There are other advanced and specialized trainings available for music therapists who would like to specialize in different areas including Guided Imagery in Music (GIM),[125] Sound Birthing,[126] and Hospice Palliative Care Music Therapy.[127] As a result, all music therapists work in their own unique way, myself included. This is similar to the many different approaches and philosophies of counselling and verbal therapies. There are also music therapists who have dedicated their whole careers working with one population or diagnosis and thus are much more specialised in that particular field than I am. However, this book is simply full of memorable stories from my experiences that I wanted to share. I hope you enjoyed reading this book as much as I enjoyed telling the stories. I also hope you have been as inspired by these stories as I have been while experiencing them.

We can never escape music. It is all around us in our daily lives in supermarkets, elevators, restaurants and public transport, from the beat of a basketball to raindrops on a window. What is amazing is that, like all art, everyone has very different subjective experiences with music. Even the way we listen to music differs from person to person. Some listen to only the lyrics and don't listen to the melody or instrumentation; some listen only to the music and have no idea what any of the lyrics were after listening. Some people respond more to sad music, some heavy metal, some more to a ballad or love song. Some feel indifferent about music and some don't like listening to music at all. But what is certain is that music touches us all at some point in our lives and we all use music in very different ways. We often turn to music when we don't have the words to express our feelings. It can be what we crave when we're celebrating, when we're grieving, when we're falling in love. Music makes horror movies suspenseful and makes us tear up at weddings. It connects us to other people and in the words of Fearne Cotton:

> *"Music is one of the easiest ways to connect with something bigger than us."*[128]
> - Fearne Cotton, from her book Bigger Than Us

I would love it if you also wanted to connect with me!

Via social media: @gillian_cunnison

Or through my website: www.telemedmusic.com

I have also been in the fortunate position to set up my own private practice, Telemed Music, this past year.

Telemed Music provides telehealth music therapy services and adaptive lessons. I created Telemed Music because I am passionate that everyone should have access to music therapy services, even those in remote areas who are not near a music therapist, for those who may not have a means of transport or a caregiver to take them to therapy or those who find it difficult to leave their house. Furthermore, I have worked with many patients in different locations who would have significantly benefited from continuing services or perhaps even connecting with others diagnosed with the same condition and facing the same difficulties at that chapter in their lives. Now, with the wonders of technology, they can do that—even thousands of miles apart! I love the ease of this method of communication and how a simple connection can help people get through a tough time. In addition, if I can name three positive things I learned from pandemic times, it is (1) to think outside the box, (2) nothing is impossible and (3) overall, telehealth has proven to be very effective for music therapy. If you prefer in-person sessions for you or your loved one, Telemed Music can connect you with an in-person therapist.

Adaptive lessons are for learners requiring a little extra help, taught with my background training and clinical experience. I strive to help each student feel successful when learning the instrument and enjoy the experience rather than make it a chore. In addition to acquiring the skills to play an instrument and enjoy music, each student will also have the opportunity to improve receptive language skills, increase sustained attention and impulse control, develop their musicality and encourage self-expression through improvisation and composition.

You can visit my website www.telemedmusic.com to find out more!

RESOURCE LIST

Below is a list of some websites and other resources if you are interested in learning more about music therapy, some of which are mentioned throughout the book.

My Private Practice

Telemed Music - Providing virtual music therapy sessions and adaptive lessons. I would also love to talk with you about anything music therapy related—don't hesitate to reach out! www.telemedmusic.com

Music Therapy Information Websites

World Federation for Music Therapy (WFMT) - An organisation dedicated to bringing together music therapy associations and individuals interested in developing and promoting music therapy globally. Visit their website to find information about the music therapy associations of different countries worldwide. www.wfmt.info

European Music Therapy Confederation (EMTC) - Provides information on the profession and connects music therapy associations from all over Europe. www.emtc-eu.com

American Music Therapy Association (AMTA) - A 501(c)3 non-profit organisation whose mission is to advance public awareness of the benefits of music therapy and increase access to quality music therapy services in the US. AMTA works to support and strengthen the music therapy profession, expand access to music therapy, raise awareness about its benefits, support research and empower music therapists to serve diverse populations. www.musictherapy.org

British Association for Music Therapy (BAMT) - The professional body for music therapists in the UK, providing practitioners and non-practitioners with information, professional support and training opportunities. The BAMT is also dedicated to promoting and raising awareness of music therapy and providing information to the general public. www.bamt.org

Certification Board for Music Therapists (CBMT) - Awards board certification by examination for music therapists practicing in the US based on proven, up-to-date knowledge and competence in clinical practice. www.cbmt.org

Health and Care Professions Council (HCPC) - Regulator of health and care professions in the UK. By law, music therapists must register with the HCPC to practice in the UK. www.hcpc-uk.org

Nordoff & Robbins - The UK's largest music therapy charity providing music therapy and community music services across the UK. www.nordoff-robbins.org.uk

Nordoff-Robbins Center for Music Therapy - Part of New York University, the centre provides a variety of services including individual music therapy, group music therapy sessions and music instruction for people of all ages in Manhattan, NYC. https://steinhardt.nyu.edu/nordoff

The Academy of Neurologic Music Therapy - A 501(c) non-profit organisation to disseminate information about the evidence-based practice of NMT and provide opportunities for professional development in NMT that ensure best practice in the field. www.nmtacademy.co

Other Supportive Organisations

American Patriot Music Project - Provides music support for veterans through musical instrument donations, guitar-building workshops and other project support. www.americanpatriotmusic.org

Amy Winehouse Foundation - Providing music therapy services, resilience programs, recovery housing and pathways for young women and young people. www.amywinehousefoundation.org

Camp Happy Days - Providing week-long residential camps in South Carolina for children with cancer and their siblings. www.camphappydays.org

Chiltern Music Therapy - Non-profit providing music therapy, neurologic music therapy and community music services across England. www.chilternmusictherapy.co.uk

DrumSTRONG - Community organisation based in Charlotte, North Carolina, drumming to beat cancer. www.drumstrong.org

Ukulele Kids Club - Provides free ukuleles to children in hospitals as well as online resources and song sheets. www.theukc.org

Wounded Warrior Project - Provides direct programs in mental health, career counselling and long-term rehabilitative care along with advocacy efforts to improve the lives of millions of veterans and their families. www.woundedwarriorproject.org

Also, a shout out to the hundreds of celebrities and musicians who support music therapy through the Nordoff-Robbins O2 Silver Clef Awards. Including a special shoutout to my favourite band, Muse!

Instruments and Adaptive Aids

Below are some of my favourite lesser-known music therapy instruments and helpful adaptive aids I have used over the years.

Adaptive Mallets/Sticks - Various adaptive mallets, drumsticks and adaptive cuffs are available online at www.westmusic.com and other worldwide music retailers

Boomwhackers® - Colourful hollow plastic tubes tuned to a musical pitch by length. www.boomwhackers.com

Chord Buddy® - a revolutionary device that affixes to the neck of the guitar with each button creating a different chord structure. www.chordbuddy.com

Idiopan™ - A metal tongue drum that can be tuned to many different scales through a unique magnet system providing warm, rich, pure tones. www.idiopan.com

Q Chord - an accessible instrument incorporating technology from a basic keyboard and electric guitar, combining both in a portable casing with a strum plate, a rhythm section and a chord button section. Available to buy on various different websites.

Rockstix™ - Motion-activated LED light-up multi-colour change drumsticks. www.powerstix.io

ZeroGravity Orbit Guitar Pick - an adaptive pick that wraps around the thumb, making the pick easier to grasp. Available to buy on various different websites.

Documentaries

Alive Inside: A Story of Music and Memory - A 2014 documentary by Michael Rossato-Bennett "featuring interviews with family members who have witnessed the miraculous effects of music on their loved ones and experts, including renowned neurologist and best-selling author Oliver Sacks (also quoted in this book) and musician Bobby McFerrin". The full-length documentary is available on YouTube.

The Beat of the Heart - Documenting the work of music therapist Brian Schreck, the creator of the heartbeat recording technology mentioned in Chapter 10. The full-length documentary is available on Vimeo.

The Music in You - from the docuseries *Instrumental Health* by filmmaker Pete Eliot. Parts 9-12 from the docuseries focus on Nordoff-Robbins music therapy. All parts of the docuseries are available on YouTube.

Online Music Therapy Journals

Voices: A World Forum for Music Therapy (open access) - www.voices.no

British Journal of Music Therapy (restricted & open access) - http://journals.sagepub.com/home/bjmb

Journal of Music Therapy (restricted & open access) - www.academic.oup.com/jmt

Music Therapy Perspectives (restricted & open access) - https://academic.oup.com/mtp

Nordic Journal of Music Therapy (restricted & open access) - www.tandfonline.com/rnjm20

Books

Music Therapy Handbook - Edited by Barbara L. Wheeler, Ph.D., MT-BC. A comprehensive overview of music therapy, from basic concepts to emerging clinical approaches.

Handbook of Neurologic Music Therapy - Edited by Michael H. Thaut, Ph.D., MT-BC and Dr Volker Hoemberg, M.D. A text presenting each of the Neurologic Music Therapy techniques described in detail including specific exercises and pertinent background information regarding research and clinical diagnoses.

Music Therapy: Intimate Notes – Mercédès Pavlicevic. Stories and reflections describing powerful encounters between nine music therapists and their clients.

Musicophilia: Tales of Music and the Brain - Oliver Sacks, CBE, FRCP. Dr Sacks explores the place music occupies in the brain and how it affects the human condition.

Sing You Home - Jodi Picoult. A novel following the life events of the main character Zoe who is a Berklee College of Music trained music therapist.

The Music Instinct: How Music Words and Why We Can't Do Without It - Phillip Ball. A comprehensive, accessible survey of what is known and what is unknown about how music works its magic.

This is Your Brain on Music: The Science of a Human Obsession - Daniel J. Levitin, FRSC. The author, a rocker-turned-neuroscientist, explores the connection between music—its performance, its composition, how we listen to it, why we enjoy it—and the human brain.

Music Therapy Assessment Tools

Examples of music therapy assessment tools are listed in the resources below.

List of Tests and Measures Used in Music Therapy developed by Gustavo Schulz Gattino from Aalborg University. https://vbn.aau.dk/files/449332775/List_of_tests_and_measures_in_music_therapy_.docx

Music Therapy Star™ The Outcomes Star for Children Accessing Music Therapy. Developed by Triangle and Coram, 2011. https://www.outcomesstar.org.uk/using-the-star/see-the-stars/music-therapy-star/

Music Therapy Session Assessment Scale (MT-SAS): Validation of a new tool for music therapy process evaluation researched by Raglio, A., Gnesi, M., Monti, M.C., Oasi, O., Gianotti, M., Attardo, L., Gontero, G., Morotti, L., Boffelli, S., Imbriani, C., Montomoli, C., Imbriani, M. in The *Journal of Clinical Psychology & Psychotherapy.* 2017 Nov;24(6)

ACKNOWLEDGEMENTS

First and foremost, I extend my deepest gratitude to the wonderful individuals and their families who gave me permission to tell their stories.

Thank you to you, the reader, for reading my first book! And thank you to those who have shared my book with others.

The biggest thank you to my parents for always encouraging me and providing me with every opportunity to allow me to get to where I am today including learning music and pursuing further education.

Thank you to my friends and family who have encouraged me along the way and to everyone who checked in on me and held me accountable in the very long three-plus-year process of writing. I began this book without any knowledge of writing or publishing a book. In short, I had no clue what I was doing and made it up as I went along so I am just happy I eventually finished and published it! It far exceeded the amount of time and work that I thought it was going to take. The only thing I knew throughout the process was that I had stories to tell and would eventually finish them one day. I am very thankful to have had the time to be able to write this book in the first place, something which many people do not have the luxury or opportunity to do.

Thank you to Allyson, Barbara, Bryan L., Carolyn, Chris, Christina, Daciay, Dean, Elise, Gavin, Jaime, Julie, Kirsten, Kurtis, Linda, Linzi, Lizzie, Melissa, Michele, Mum, Natalie, Ryan, Sophia, Sophie and Victoria who also looked over sections and chapters. I am so grateful to you all for your support. Thank you also to Gio for being patient while I spent hundreds of hours on my laptop!

A big thank you to all my co-workers who I would have been completely lost without over the years. They are all selfless individuals and the true definition of the caring profession. Thank you Ali, Allie, Alison, Amanda, Andrea, Anna-Catherine, Anneliese, Ariel, Ashley, Becky, Betsey, Bri, Caitlin C., Caitlin H.P, Carli, Carolina, Chelsea, Chrissy, Christina, Courtney, Dana, Danae, Dani, Danielle, Dean, Elizabeth K., Elizabeth R., Ellen, Emily, Eric, Fred, Gretchen, Hannah, Heather, Hailey, Helen, Hunter, Jack, Jamie L.P., Jen, Jenn B., Jenn G., Jenna B., Jenna H., Jeri B., Jill, Jim, John, Julie L., Julie P., Julie W., Kathleen, Kelly, Keri, Kerri L.M., Kerri S.C., Kim, Kirsten, Kristen K., Kristin, Laura F., Laura P, Laura T., Lauren M., Lauren P., Laurie, Leslie, Lisa C., Lisa L., Mackinley, Madi, Maddy, Maggie, Mary, Mason, Matt, Meg S.J., Meg W., Megan, Meghan C., Meghan E., Melinda, Melissa, Meredith, Michelle C., Michelle H., Mike, Molly, Morgan, Moriah, Rita, Roberta, Robin, Roia, Rose, Rosemary, Sadie, Sara Jane, Sara, Sarah C., Sarah F., Sarah N.L., Shannon, Sharon, Sheri, Stacey, Stephanie K., Stephanie S., Terri and Varvara. To all the students I have supervised over the years, thank you for helping me grow and learn too!

Thank you to my bandmates too over the years including Amy, Andrew, Anna, Ben, Bradly, Calum, Charlie, Chiron, Cody, Daciay, David, Derek, Dez, Emanuel, Ethan, Fred D., Fred H., Geoff, Gersh, Jack, Jason, Jay, Jeff, Jim, Joe, Josh, Julie, Kat, Kelsey, Kevin, Kyle, Lauren, Liam, Lizzie, Louisa, Luke, Mark, Max, Michael, Moira, Molly, Nadia, Natalie, Nicky, Patrick, Paul, Paula, Rob, Rhys, Richard, Rob, Sam, Selina, Shaun, Shona, Spiro, Steven C., Steven H., Susan, Tasha, Travis, Tim, Todd, Tyler and Zak. You all rock!

Thank you to my friends in my master's degree program—Lizzie, Juliette, Laura, Gráinne, Rachel and Debbie, without whom I wouldn't have made it through to become a music therapist in the first place. I am thankful for your support and friendship. So many hours together and so many cups of tea! My first supervisor, Gill and my professors, James, Emma and April—thank you for your knowledge and guidance. Thank you to my brother Ross, who generously contributed towards the high cost of my master's degree. Thank you to Seamus, who guided me through the long and challenging process of becoming board-certified in the United States, to Julie and Melissa for your generosity in agreeing to supervise me in Fort Myers, and to Patrick for showing me around CHOP and fuelling my passion for work in children's hospitals all those years ago.

Thank you to the authors who provided helpful free seminars and resources for first-time writers, including Alexa Bigwarfe, Chandler Bolt, Gillian Perkins, Jerry Jenkins,

Matt Rud and Morgan Gist McDonald. You definitely helped me navigate this big, scary world of writing and publishing!

Thank you to all the music therapists worldwide who are doing amazing work with countless individuals and spreading the word about music therapy. Thanks also to all the advocating music therapists, including all the state task forces in the United States, especially the dedicated Dr Kimberly Sena Moore and Dr Dena Register.

Finally and most importantly, I am eternally grateful and appreciative of every individual I have been fortunate to work with over the years. You are why we do what we do and what makes music therapy so powerful.

REFERENCES

Author's Note

1. *1.6 Respect and protect the client's confidentiality at all times and following any applicable institutional or legal rules and regulations*, from: "American Music Therapy Association Code of Ethics." *American Music Therapy Association,* updated Nov 2019, https://www.musictherapy.org/about/ethics/

2. Referenced from King, Betsey. Music Heard So Deeply: A Music Therapy Memoir. Booklocker.com, 2015.

Introduction

3. Dessen, Sarah. *Just Listen*. Viking Press, 2006.

4. "The History of Music Therapy." *American Music Therapy Association*. www.musictherapy.org/about/history. Accessed October 12, 2022.

5. Heppenheimer, T.A. "The Oldest Oldies: Caveman Music. Science & Medicine." *The LA Times*. December 23, 1991. www.latimes.com/archives/la-xpm-1991-12-23-me-608-story.html

6. "Music Therapy and Military Populations: A Status Report and Recommendations on Music Therapy Treatment, Programs, Research, and Practice Policy." *American Music Therapy Association,* 2014. www.musictherapy.org/assets/1/7/MusicTherapyMilitaryPops_2014.pdf

7. "What is Music Therapy?" *American Music Therapy Association*. www.musictherapy.org/about/musictherapy. Accessed March 23, 2022.

8   Tommasini. Anthony. "A Jazz Pianist Flips Bach Upside-Down". *The New York Times,* May 15, 2020. www.nytimes.com/2020/05/15/arts/music/dan-tepfer-bach.html

Chapter 1: I Am a Crocodile

9   "Discover Music: Hans Christian Andersen". *Classic FM.* www.classicfm.com/discover-music/latest/quotes-about-classical-music/andersen. Accessed October 15, 2023.

10 "Steel Drum Blues Scale Record Attempt #1". YouTube, uploaded by Danny the Steel Pan Drummer, Feb 5, 2023, https://www.youtube.com/watch?v=p62MckoTMEc

11 "Steven Wiltshire Draws New York." *Steven Wiltshire.* www.stephenwiltshire.co.uk/new-york-skyline-panorama. Accessed November 18, 2022.

12 Reynolds, Eileen. "What Can Music Do? Rethinking Autism Through Music Therapy." *NYU News*, New York University, modified July 22, 2016. www.nyu.edu/about/news-publications/news/2016/july/autism-and-neurodiversity-at-nordoff-robbins-center-for-music-th.html

13 Ibid

14 Gascho-White, Wanda. "'The Music Child'—the Role of Music Therapy in the Over-all Treatment Plan for Special Needs Children." *Communicative Disorders Assistant Association of Canada.* www.cdaac.ca/wp-content/uploads/2015/12/resources_The-Music-Child.pdf. Accessed October 15, 2023.

15 Reynolds, Eileen. "What Can Music Do? Rethinking Autism Through Music Therapy."

16 Aigen, Kenneth. "Music-Centered Dimensions of Nordoff-Robbins Music Therapy." *Music Therapy Perspectives*, Vol 32, Issue 1 pp.18-29, June 23, 2014.

17 Reynolds, Eileen. "What Can Music Do? Rethinking Autism Through Music Therapy".

18 Levitin, Daniel J. *This is Your Brain on Music: The Science of a Human Obsession.* Penguin Press, 2006.

19　"Why Don't We Stutter When We Sing?" *Stuttering Treatment and Research Trust (START).* https://www.stuttering.co.nz/news/why-dont-we-stutter-when-we-sing/. Accessed June 14, 2023.

20　"Alignment Principles: Kinaesthetic Awareness". NSW Education Standards Authority. https://sites.google.com/education.nsw.gov.au/hscdance/core-performance/alignment-principles/kinaesthetic-awareness. Accessed October 30, 2023.

21　Dukes, Greg. "Frisson: Why Music Can Give You Chills or Goosebumps." *BBC Reels*, British Broadcasting Corporation, January 19, 2023. https://www.bbc.com/reel/playlist/a-sensory-world?vpid=p0dhymc0

22　Explained: Music. Directed by Joe Postner, Vox Media, 2018.

23　Che, Y., Jicol, C., Ashwin, C. *et al.* "An RCT study showing few weeks of music lessons enhance audio-visual temporal processing". *Nature Scientific Reports,* vol. 12: 20087, November 22, 2022.

24　Cahart, M.-S., Amad, A., Draper, S. B., Lowry, R. G., Marino, L., Carey, C., Ginestet, C. E., Smith, M. S., & Williams, S. C. R. "The Effect of Learning to Drum on Behavior and Brain Function in Autistic Adolescents". *Proceedings of the National Academy of Sciences,* vol. 119 No. 23. June 7, 2022.

25　Ibid

Chapter 2: Ring of Fire

26　"Definition and Quotes About Music Therapy". American Music Therapy Association. https://www.musictherapy.org/about/quotes/. Accessed November 1, 2023.

27　Brown, Jeffrey & Davenport, Anne Azzi. "How Gabby Giffords is using music to rewire her brain after being shot." *PBS News Hour, Newshour Productions LLC*, April 8, 2021. www.pbs.org/newshour/show/how-gabby-giffords-is-using-music-to-rewire-her-brain-after-being-shot

28　Conklyn, D., Novak, E., Boissy, A., Bethoux, F., & Chemal, K. "The Effects of Modified Melodic Intonation Therapy on Non-Fluent Aphasia: A Pilot Study." *Journal of Speech, Language and Hearing Research.* EPublication, March 12, 2012.

29   Ouellette, Joy. "The Effect of a Rhythmic Speech Cuing Protocol on Speech Intelligibility in Patients with Parkinson's Disease". *University of Miami, Masters Thesis.* September 15, 2015. https://scholarship.miami.edu/esploro/outputs/graduate/The-Effect-of-a-Rhythmic-Speech/991031447673902976

30   Edited by Thaut, Michael. H. and Hoemberg, Volker. 2014. *Handbook of Neurologic Music Therapy.* Oxford University Press, 2014.

Chapter 3: I Believe

31   Simpson, Porsche. "Interview: Unparalleled Talent Kelly Price is Back for More". *Parlé Magazine.* March 2011. www.parlemag.com/2011/03/unparalleled-talent-kelly-price-is-back-for-more/

32   Bates, D., Bolwell, B., Majhail, N.S., Rybicki, L., Yurch, M., Abounader, D., Kohuth, J., Jarancik, S., Koniarczyk, H., McLellan, L., Dabney, J., Lawrence, C., Gallagher, L., Kalaycio, M., Sobecks, R., Dean, R., Hill, B., Pohlman, B., Hamilton, B.K., Gerds, A.T., Jagadeesh, D., Liu, H.D. "Music Therapy for Symptom Management After Autologous Stem Cell Transplantation: Results From a Randomized Study". *Biology of Blood Marrow Transplantation,* vol. 9 pp.1567-1572. September 23, 2017.

33   Stanczyk, Malgorzata Monika. "Music therapy in supportive cancer care". *Reports of Practical Oncology & Radiotherapy*, vol. 16(5):170-2, June 8, 2011.

34   Ball, Phillip. *The Music Instinct: How Music Works and Why We Can't Do Without It.* Oxford University Press, 2012 p.245.

35   Rossetti, A., Chadha, M., Torres, B.N., Lee, J.K., Hylton, D., Loewy, J.V., Harrison, L.B. "The Impact of Music Therapy on Anxiety in Cancer Patients Undergoing Simulation for Radiation Therapy". *International Journal of Radiation, Oncology, Biology and Physics,* vol. 99 Issue 1, pp.103-110. September 1, 2017.

36   Davis, William B., Gfeller, Kate E. and Thaut, Michael H. *An Introduction to Music Therapy, Theory and Practice.* The American Music Therapy Association, 2008.

Chapter 4: When the Saints Go Marching In

37   Sheffield, Rob. *Talking to Girls About Duran Duran: One Young Man's Quest for True Love and a Cooler Haircut.* Penguin Press, 2010.

38 Kelechi, T.J., Muise-Helmericks, R.C., Theeke, L.A., Cole, S.W., Madisetti, M., Mueller, M., Prentice, M.A. "An observational study protocol to explore loneliness and systemic inflammation in an older adult population with chronic venous leg ulcers". *BMC Geriatrics*, vol. 21 Issue 1, p.118. February 10, 2021.

39 "George Harrison - The Early Years". *Mail Online, The Daily Mail.* www.dailymail.co.uk/news/article-87098/George-Harrison--The-early-years.html. Accessed 28 October, 2022.

40 Cotton, Fearne. *Bigger than Us.* EBury Press, 2022.

41 "Music and Health". *Harvard Health Publishing - Harvard Medical School.* September 11, 2021. https://www.health.harvard.edu/newsletter_article/music-and-health

42 Fancourt, D. & Williamon, A. "Attending a concert reduces glucocorticoids, progesterone and the cortisol/DHEA ratio". *Journal of Public Health*, vol. 132 pp.101-104. March 2016.

43 Ibid

44 Patrick Fagan et al. "Science says gig-going can help you live longer and increases well-being". *Virgin Media O2,* March 27, 2018. https://news.virginmedia02.co.uk/archive/science-says-gig-going-can-help-you-live-longer-and-increases-wellbeing/

45 "Interview #112 – Pete Townshend". Interviewed by John Gilliland for *Pop Chronicles Radio Series*, February 5, 1968. https://digital.library.unt.edu/ark:/67531/metadc1692078/?q=pop%20chronicles%20pete%20townshend

Chapter 5: Always a Star That Shines

46 Austin Steve. "When Your Mental Illness Comes in Waves". *The Mighty.* November 9, 2022. www.themighty.com/topic/anxiety/anxiety-depression-comes-in-waves/

47 Kestel, Dévora. "The State of Mental Health Globally in the Wake of the COVID-19 Pandemic and Progress on the WHO Special Initiative for Mental Health (2019-2023)". *UN Chronicle, United Nations.* October 10, 2022. www.un.org/en/un-chronicle/state-mental-health-globally-wake-covid-19-pandemic-and-progress-who-special-initiative

48 Bridge, J. A., Ruch, D. A., Sheftall, A. H., Hahm, H. C., O'Keefe, V. M., Fontanella, C. A., Brock, G., Campo, J. V., & Horowitz, L. M. "Youth suicide during the first year of the COVID-19 pandemic". *Journal of Pediatrics*, vol. 151 Issue 3. February 15, 2023.

49 Gaylor, E.M., Krause, K.H., Welder, L.E., et al. "Suicidal Thoughts and Behaviors Among High School Students—Youth Risk Behavior Survey", *CDC United States,* 2021. 72:45–54.

50 Brownlee, Shannon and Garber, Judith. "Overprescribed: High Cost isn't America's Only Drug Problem". *First Opinion: Boston Globe Media.* April 2, 2019. www.statnews.com/2019/04/02/overprescribed-americas-other-drug-problem

51 Erikson, Erik H. *Identity, Youth and Crisis.* W.W. Norton Company, 1968.

52 Shipley, A. and Odell-Miller, H. "The Role of Music Therapy for Anxious Adolescent School Refusers: The Importance of Identity". *The British Journal of Music Therapy*, vol. 26 No. 1. June 12, 2012.

53 Ibid

54 Ibid

55 "Outburst". *Base 51.* www.base51.org/outburst. Accessed 24 April, 2023.

56 "A Place Where I Could Meet Other LGBT People - Reece's Story". *National Foundation for Youth Music.* https://youthmusic.org.uk/reeces-story. Accessed February 12, 2023.

57 Yerushalmi, Hanoch. 2007. Paradox and personal growth during crisis. *The American Journal of Psychoanalysis*, vol. 67 issue 4, pp.359-380. December 2007./

58 Shipley, A. and Odell-Miller, H. "The Role of Music Therapy for Anxious Adolescent School Refusers: The Importance of Identity".

59 Pasiali, V., D. Quick, J. Hassall, and H. A. Park. "Music Therapy Programming for Persons With Eating Disorders: A Review With Clinical Examples". *Voices: A World Forum for Music Therapy*, vol. 20, no. 3, October 30, 2020, p. 15

60 Thambirajah, M.S. et al. *Understanding School Refusal.* Jessica Kingsley Publishers, 2008.

Chapter 6: Sympathy for the Devil

61 *"One on One: Interview with David Bowie". Livewire,* June 16, 2022. http://www.concertlivewire.com/interviews/bowie.htm

62 Karageorghis, C. I., Priest, D. L., Williams, L. S., Hirani, R. M., Lannon, K. M., & Bates, B. J. "Ergogenic and psychological effects of synchronous music during circuit-type exercise". *Journal of Psychology of Sport and Exercise,* vol. 11 issue 6, pp.551–559. June 25, 2010.

63 Jabr, Ferris. "Let's Get Physical: The Psychology of Effective Workout Music". *Scientific American.* March 20, 2013. www.scientificamerican.com/article/psychology-workout-music/

64 Sills, D. and Todd, A. "Does Music Directly Affect a Person's Heart Rate?" *Medical Education Faculty Publications, Wright State University.* February 4, 2015. www.corescholar.libraries.wright.edu/cgi/viewcontent.cgi?article=1000&context=med_education

65 Bradt, J., Magee, W.L., Dileo, C., Wheeler, B.L., McGilloway, E. "Music therapy for acquired brain injury". *Cochrane Database of Systematic Reviews* Issue 7. January 20, 2017.

66 Hogue, J.D. "NMT Pictochart". https://create.piktochart.com/output/4062942-untitled-infographic. Accessed 11th December, 2022.

67 Magee, W.L. "Why include music in a neuro-rehabiliation team?" *Journal for Advances in Clinical Neuroscience and Rehabilitation.* Vol. 19, No. 2. 2020. October 1, 2019.

68 "MedRhythms Announces FDA Listing of InTandem™(MR-001) to Improve Walking and Ambulation in Adults with Chronic Stroke". *PRNewswire,* July 6, 2023. www.prnewswire.com/news-releases/medrhythms-announces-fda-listing-of-intandem-mr-001-to-improve-walking-and-ambulation-in-adults-with-chronic-stroke-301871199.html

69 Oliver Sacks, *Musicophilia: Tales of Music and the Brain.* Vintage Books, 2008.

Chapter 7: Stand Tall

70 Kaur, Rabjir. "Music". Pinterest.com. https://in.pinterest.com/pin/644929609143101776. Accessed September 28, 2023.

71 "Briefing: Adoption of Children in the European Union". *European Parliament.* June 2016. https://www.europarl.europa.eu/RegData/etudes/BRIE/2016/583860/EPRS_BRI(2016)583860_EN.pdf

72 Petrowski N, Cappa C, & Gross P. "Estimating the number of children in formal alternative care: Challenges and results". *Journal of Child Abuse and Neglect,* vol. 70, pp.388-398. Jun 1, 2017

73 Lefevre, Michelle. 2004. "Playing with sound: The therapeutic use of music in direct work with children". *Child and Family Social Work E-Journal, vol.* 9 Issue 4, p.340

74 Ibid

75 King, Betsey. *Music Therapy: Another path to learning and communication for children on the autistic spectrum.* p.6. Future Horizons Inc., 2004.

76 Odell-Miller, Helen. "Value of music therapy for people with personality disorders". *Journal of Mental Health Practice*, vol.14, Issue 1 p.34. July 3, 2011.

77 Chiang, Jenny Yu Kuan. "Music Therapy for Young Children who have special needs: The music therapy experience from the perspectives of carers and professionals". *New Zealand School of Music, Masters Thesis,* p.10. November 5, 2010.

78 Fong, Christina Ting. "The Effects of Emotional Ambivalence on Creativity". *The Academy of Management Journal*, vol. 49(5), pp.1016–1030. October, 2006.

79 Pasiali, Varvara. "Resilience, music therapy, and human adaption: nurturing young children and families". *Nordic Journal of Music Therapy,* vol. 21, Issue 1, p.46. July 9, 2011.

Chapter 8: Oh, What a Beautiful Mornin'

80 Schroeder, Lisa. *Chasing Brooklyn.* Simon & Schuster, 2011.

81 "Alzheimer's Disease Facts and Figures". *Alzheimer's Association.* 2023. https://www.alz.org/media/Documents/alzheimers-facts-and-figures.pdf

82 "What is Dementia?" *National Health Service (NHS).* Reviewed 20 July 2023. https://www.nhs.uk/conditions/dementia/about-dementia/what-is-dementia

83 "FDA Converts Novel Alzheimer's Disease Treatment to Traditional Approval". *US Food & Drug Administration*. July 6, 2023. www.fda.gov/news-events/press-announcements/fda-converts-novel-alzheimers-disease-treatment-traditional-approval

84 Jacobsen, J.-H., Stelzer, J., Hans Fritz, T., Chételat, G., La Joie, R., Turner, R. "Why musical memory can be preserved in advanced Alzheimer's disease". Brain: A Journal of Neurology. Vol. 138, Issue 8, pp. 2438–2450. August 2015.

85 "Songs to Listen to During Mental Health Awareness Month". *Jinx*. May 9, 2022. www.moonstar2016.wordpress.com/2022/05/09

86 "Listening to music could improve memory for older patients". *Spectrum News One, Charter Communications*. September 6, 2022. https://spectrumlocalnews.com/nc/charlotte/health/2022/08/30/listening-to-music-could-improve-memory-for-other-patients

87 Quinci, M.A., Belden, A., Goutama, V. et al. Longitudinal changes in auditory and reward systems following receptive music-based intervention in older adults. Journal of Scientific Reports 12, Article no. 11517, July 7, 2022.

88 King, J.B., Jones, K.G., Goldberg, E., Rollins, M., MacNamee, K., Moffit, C., Naidu, S.R., Ferguson, M.A., Garcia-Leavitt, E., Amaro, J., Breitenbach, K.R., Watson, J.M., Gurgel, R.K., Anderson, J.S., Foster, N.L. "Increased Functional Connectivity After Listening to Favored Music in Adults With Alzheimer Dementia". The Journal of Prevention of Alzheimer's Disease, Vol. 6 Issue 1 pp.56-62. Jan 1, 2019.

89 United States Congress. *S.1723 - 102nd Congress. Music Therapy for Older Americans Act*. September 24, 1991. www.congress.gov/bill/102nd-congress/senate-bill/1723

90 Branson, Jenny L. "Leaving the Profession: A Grounded Theory Exploration of Music Therapists' Decisions". *Voices: A World Forum for Music Therapy*, Vol. 23 Issue 1. March 3, 2023.

91 Roy, Aishwarya. "Music and Memories". *Orange Diary*. May 27, 2022. https://imtnagpur.wordpress.com/2022/05/27/music-and-memories/

92 "Oliver Sacks – Musicophilia – Music Therapy & Parkinson's." YouTube, uploaded by Knopfgroup, October 8, 2007. https://www.youtube.com/watch?v=9nnLTPPDRXI

93 Wasserstrom, Chuck. "Oh, Say Can They Sing: Trembling Troubadours Show Off Their Voices". *UTC News*. July 25, 2022. https://blog.utc.edu/news/2022/07/oh-say-can-they-sing-trembling-troubadours-show-off-their-voices/

94 "Study: Memories of Music cannot be lost to Alzheimer's and Dementia." Oliver Sacks Foundation. www.facebook.com/oliversacks

95 Testimonies shared with permission from both choir members

96 Thompson, J. D., Talmage, A., Jenkins, B., & Purdy, S. "Quality of Life for People who Sing: An Exploration of Participant Experiences Singing in Neurological and Community Choirs Across New Zealand." *Voices: A World Forum for Music Therapy* vol. 22, Issue 2. July 1, 2022

Chapter 9: Pain Don't Hurt Me No More

97 Hooper, Lauren Alex. "Quotes that helped me (Songwriting Edition)". *Finding Hope*, December 11, 2021. www.finding-hope.co.uk/tag/special-interests

Chapter 10: No One Like You

98 Coleman, Naomi. "Why listening to music is the key to good health". *Daily Mail*. http://www.dailymail.co.uk/health/article-137116/Why-listening-music-key-good-health.html#ixzz4nqsoOcXD. Accessed May 12, 2023.

99 "Early Brain and Child Development 101: Why Peekaboo Matters". *Harvard University Center on the Developing Child: HCDC Pediatrics*. https://pediatrics.developingchild.harvard.edu/resource/early-brain-and-child-development-101-why-peekaboo-matters. Accessed July 31, 2022.

100 "The Science of Early Childhood Development (*InBrief*)". *Center on the Developing Child: Harvard University*. 2007. Retrieved from:www.developingchild.harvard.edu.

101 Kirschner, S. & Tomasello, M. "Joint music making promotes prosocial behavior in 4-year-old children". *Journal of Evolution and Human Behavior*, Vol. 31, Issue 5, p.354. September 2010.

102 Pearce, E., Launay, J., & Dunbar, R.I. "The ice-breaker effect: Singing mediates fast social bonding". *The Royal Society: Journal of Open Science,* vol. 2 Issue 10. October 28, 2015.

103 Anshel, A. & Kipper, D.A. "The Influence of Group Singing on Trust and Cooperation". *Journal of Music Therapy*, Vol. 25, Issue 3, pp.145–155. September 1988.

104 Cole, Diane. "Your Aging Brain Will Be in Better Shape if You've Taken Music Lessons." *In Focus: National Geographic.* January 3, 2014. https://www.nationalgeographic.com/culture/article/140103-music-lessons-brain-aging-cognitive-neuroscience

105 Lamont, Alexandra. "Toddlers' musical preferences: musical preference and musical memory in the early years". *Annals of the New York Academy of Sciences: The Neurosciences and Music*, vol. 999, Issue 1. January 24, 2006.

106 Flom, R., Gentile, D.A. & Pick, A.D. "Infants' discrimination of happy and sad music". *Journal of Infant Behavior and Development*, vol. 4, pp.716-28. December 31, 2008.

107 Heart and Harmony Sound Birthing™ Music Therapy. www.heartandharmony.com

108 Joanne Loewy DA, LCAT, MT-BC on Evidence-based Use of Lullaby Ocean Disc. YouTube, uploaded by Remo Rhythm Wellness and You, July 22, 2015. https://www.youtube.com/watch?v=MWG_uM3pDGE

109 "Infant and Young Child Feeding: Model Chapter for Textbooks for Medical Students and Allied Health Professionals Session 1, The importance of infant and young child feeding and recommended practices". *World Health Organization.* 2009. https://www.ncbi.nlm.nih.gov/books/NBK148967

110 "Musical pacifier invention to help premature babies one lullaby at a time". *Florida State University News*, *Florida State University.* May 21, 2012. https://news.fsu.edu/news/arts-humanities/2012/05/21/musical-pacifier-invention-to-help-premature-babies-one-lullaby-at-a-time

111 www.lullafeed.com

112 Schreck, B., Loewy, J., LaRocca, RV., Harman, E., & Archer-Nanda, E. "Amplified Cardiopulmonary Recordings: Music Therapy Legacy Intervention with Adult Oncology Patients and Their Fam-

ilies-A Preliminary Program Evaluation". *Journal of Palliative Medicine*, vol. 25 Issue 9, pp.1409-1412. Apr 26, 2022.

113 Peterson, Mindy NCTM. "Heartbeat Music: Crafting Forever Songs of Connection; with Brian Schreck, MA, MT-BC". Enhance Life with Music Podcast. Episode 168, October 17, 2023. https://mpetersonmusic.com/podcast/episode168

114 Schreck, B. & Economos, A. "Heartbeat Recording and Composing in Perinatal Palliative Care and Hospice Music Therapy". *Journal of Music and Medicine,* Vol. 10 Issue 1 pp.22-25. January 26, 2018.

115 "Levine Children's Brings Music to Patients & Families". YouTube, uploaded by Atrium Health, October 1, 2020, www.youtube.com/watch?v=YDIZFXrRckk

116 Ibid

117 Ibid

Chapter 11: Somewhere Over the (other side of the) Rainbow

118 Juma, Norbert. "Rainbow Quotes Celebrating Hope After a Storm". *Everyday Power.* Updated October 24, 2023. https://everydaypower.com/rainbow-quotes/

119 Belland, Judy. "Why Did you Leave Music Therapy? One (ex-)Music Therapist's Answer". *Music Therapy Clinician,* Vol. 2, December 2016. https://njmusictherapy.org/wp-content/uploads/2019/08/MT-Clinician-2.pdf

120 Rafieyan, R. "So you want to become a music therapist?" *The Mindful Music Therapist Blog.* November 28, 2010. https://mindfulmusictherapist.blogspot.com/2010/11/so-you-want-to-become-music-therapist.html

121 Abrams, B. "McMusicTherapy McMarketing: Reflections Upon the Promotion of Music Therapy Services in an Increasingly Commercial Economic Climate". *Voices: A World Forum for Music Therapy*, vol. 14 Issue 2. June 24, 2014.

122 Branson, Jenny L. "Leaving the Profession: A Grounded Theory Exploration of Music Therapists' Decisions". *Voices: A World Forum for Music Therapy*, Vol. 23 Issue 1. March 3, 2023.

Chapter 12: A Note to the Trainee Music Therapist

123 Satrom, Brandon. "How I Became a Maker". *Medium, A Medium Corporation.* July 3, 2017. https://medium.com/breadboardeaux/how-i-became-a-maker-b933eee4366e

124 Kaiser, Marion. "An Exploration of Creative Arts-Based Self-Care Practices among Music Therapy Students". *Theses & Dissertations, Molly University.* 2017. https://digitalcommons.molloy.edu/cgi/viewcontent.cgi?article=1052&context=etd

Concluding Thoughts

125 Bonny Method of Guided Imagery in Music (GIM) https://music.appstate.edu/academics/special-programs/bonny-method

126 Sound Birthing https://soundbirthingmusic.com/courses/

127 Hospice & Palliative Care Therapy. https://hospicemusictherapy.org

128 Cotton, Fearne. *Bigger than Us.* EBury Press, 2022.

ABOUT THE AUTHOR

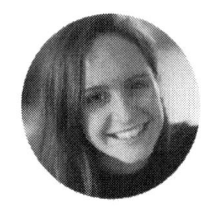

Gillian is a board-certified music therapist originally from Scotland and has spent the past decade working in many different settings across the USA including children's hospitals, an acute rehabilitation hospital, schools, memory care facilities, outpatient clinics and private practices. She has also worked as a practicum supervisor and adjunct professor at Queens University of Charlotte.

She holds a Bachelor of Arts from the University of Glasgow (2009) and a Master of Science in Music Therapy from Queen Margaret University (2013). She is a Fellow of the Academy for Neurologic Music Therapy (NMT-F) and is a Certified Brain Injury Specialist (CBIS). She holds additional certifications in DIRFloortime®, NICU Music Therapy from the National Institute for Infant & Child Medical Music Therapy and a Diploma in Percussion Performance from the Associated Board of the Royal Schools of Music. She also served for two years as an Associate Editor for the *Music Therapy Clinician* and on the New Jersey State Task Force. Gillian has played in various bands, orchestras and ensembles around the world including in the UK, US, Australia, Europe and South America.

Gillian is the owner and founder of Telemed Music, providing music therapy sessions and adaptive lessons. Visit www.telemedmusic.com for more information.

In her spare time she loves to travel, be outdoors and spend time with friends and family. Gillian loves sharing the power of music therapy with others and is very excited to have published her first book.

Gillian Cunnison

MA, MT-BC, NMT-F, NICU MT, DipABRSM

Printed in Great Britain
by Amazon